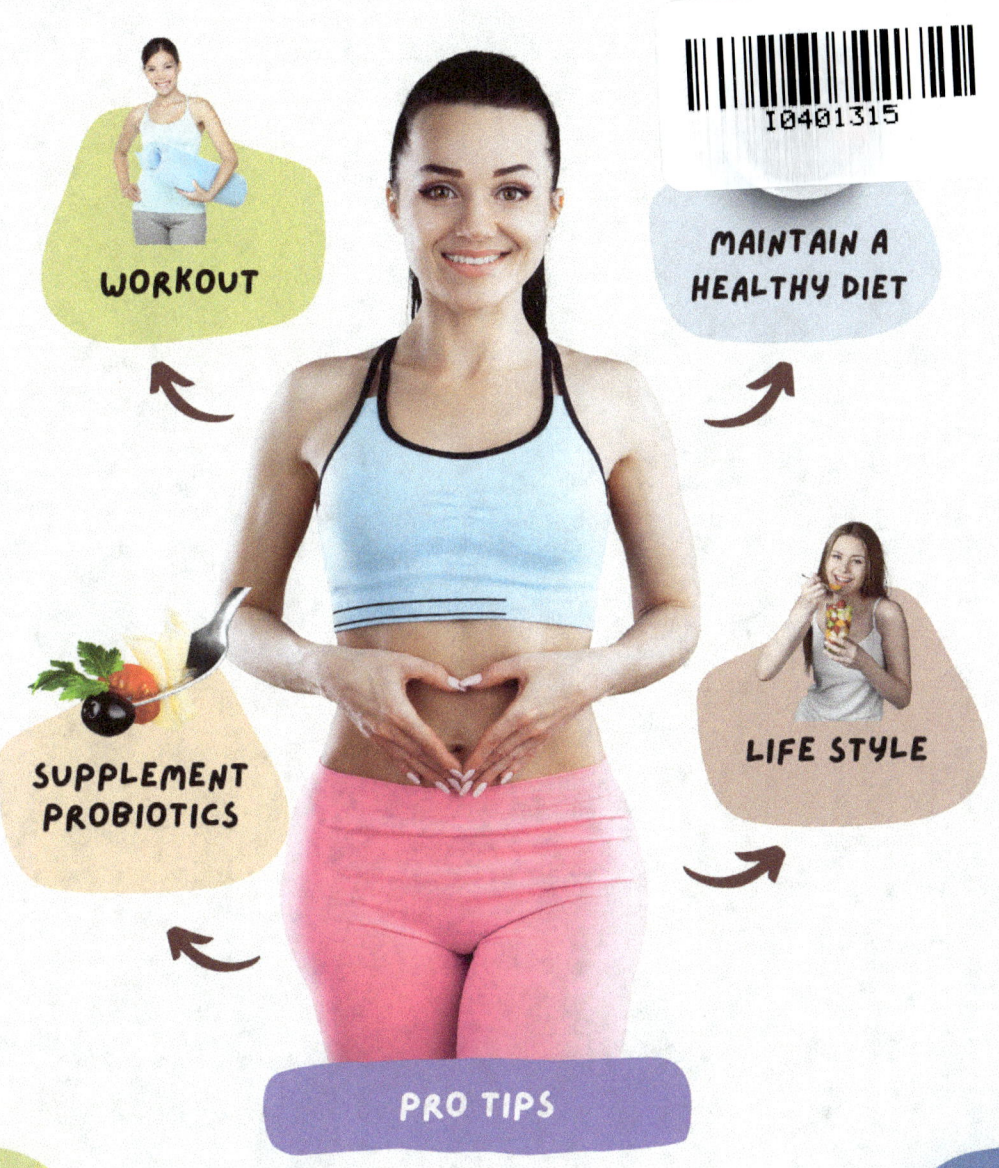

INTRODUCTION

Have you ever felt the grumble of indigestion, the discomfort of bloating, or the sluggishness that comes with irregular digestion? These common issues can be a sign of an imbalance in your gut health. But the good news is, your gut is more resilient than you might think, and with a few simple changes, you can unlock its incredible potential for improved digestion and overall well-being.

This book, "Gut Health Hacks: Simple Ways to Improve Your Digestion and Overall Well-being," is your guide to reclaiming control of your gut health. We'll delve into the fascinating world of your gut microbiome, the trillions of bacteria that reside within you and play a crucial role in digestion, immunity, and even mood. You'll learn how to identify the signs of an unhealthy gut and discover practical, science-backed hacks to nurture a thriving gut microbiome.

Forget complicated diets and restrictive lifestyles. This book focuses on small, sustainable changes you can incorporate into your daily routine. We'll explore the power of a diverse diet rich in fiber and prebiotics, the importance of hydration, and the surprising link between stress management and gut health. You'll find delicious recipes, easy-to-follow meal plans, and mindfulness practices to support your gut's journey towards optimal health.

By the end of this book, you'll be equipped with the knowledge and tools to transform your gut health. You'll experience improved digestion, increased energy levels, a stronger immune system, and a newfound sense of well-being. Are you ready to unlock the power within your gut? Let's begin!

Table content

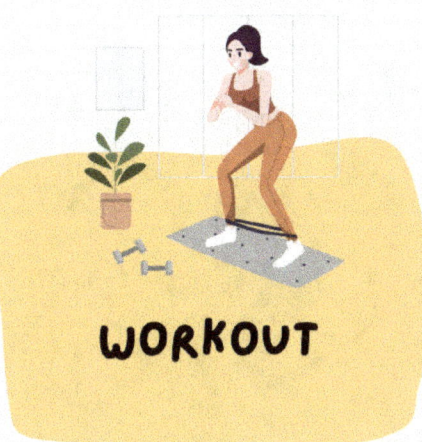

WORKOUT

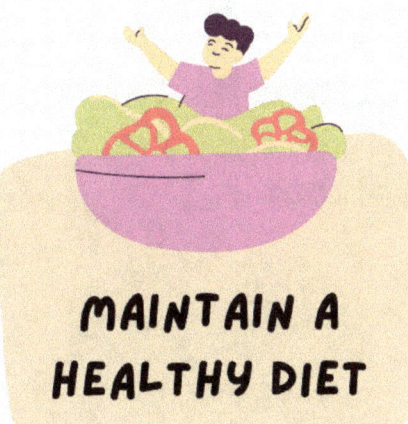

MAINTAIN A HEALTHY DIET

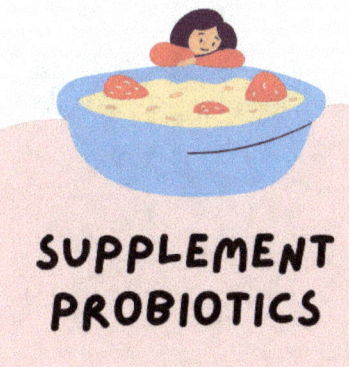

SUPPLEMENT PROBIOTICS

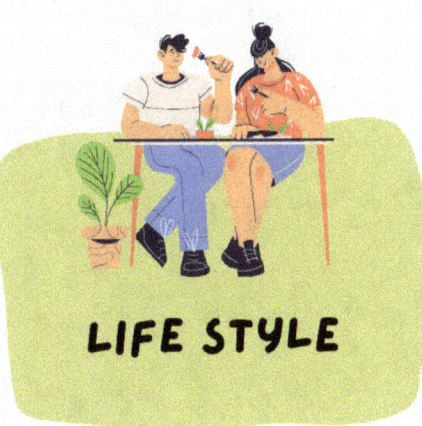

LIFE STYLE

Table of CONTENTS

Gut Health & The Microbiome — 1

Workout — 10

    Yoga — 12

    Jogging — 14

    Walking — 15

    Swimming — 16

    Cycling — 17

    Elliptical — 18

    Tai Chi — 19

    Pilates — 20

    Choose Your Exercise Plan — 22

Maintain a healthy diet — 23

Table of CONTENTS

Base your meals on higher fibre starchy carbohydrates		25
Eat lots of fruit and veg		31
Eat more fish, including a portion of oily fish		32
Cut down on saturated fat and sugar		33
Eat less salt: no more than 6g a day for adults		35

Natural Gut Health Hacks — 38

Supplement probiotics — 45

Guide to choosing the best probiotic supplements		46
Probiotic Disruptors		55
Gut-Support Hacks		58

Life style — 64

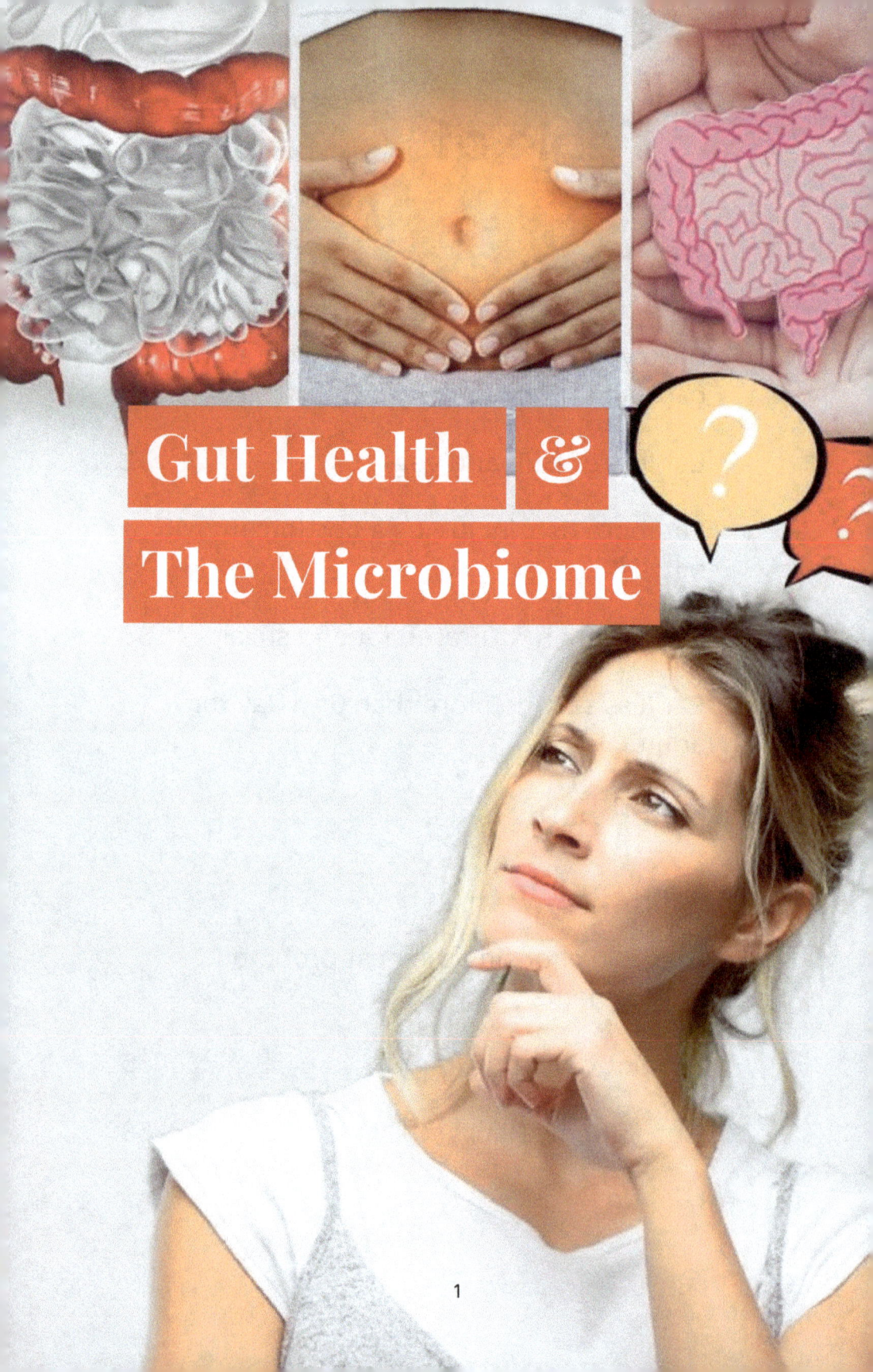

Why is the gut microbiome important to health?

The human body contains billions of different microorganisms, including fungi, bacteria, and viruses. Many types of microorganisms can cause certain diseases, including the gut microbiota which plays an extremely important role in digestion, immunity, weight, cardiovascular and many other aspects. other of health.

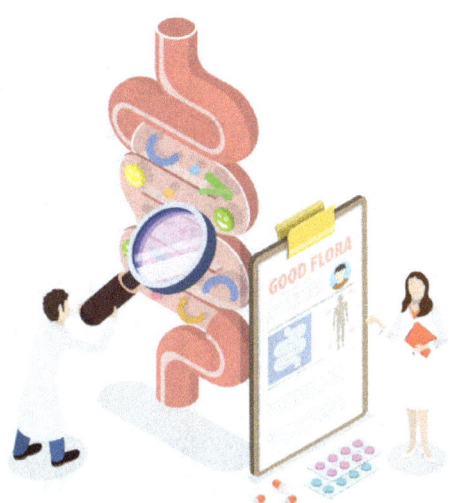

What is the gut microbiome?

Viruses, bacteria, fungi, and other microscopic living organisms are collectively known as microorganisms. In fact, there are billions of different types of microorganisms that exist on the skin and inside the intestines of the human body.

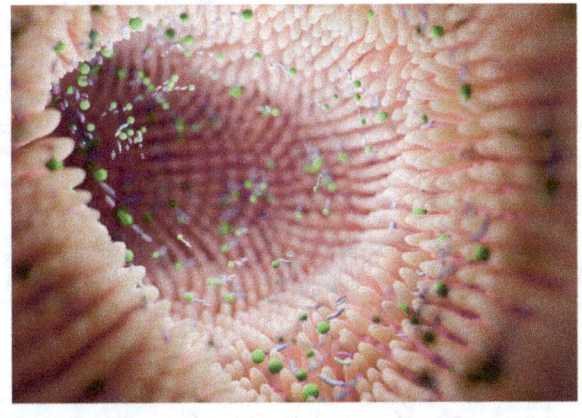

Most of the microorganisms in the intestinal tract are found in a pouch of the large intestine, called the cecum, and they are called the gut microbiota.

Although many different types of microorganisms exist inside your body, the most studied species is probably bacteria. In fact, there are more bacterial cells in your body than there are human cells. Research shows that there are about 40 trillion bacterial cells in the human body and only about 30 trillion human cells.

In particular, there are up to 1000 species of bacteria in the human gut microbiota. Each of them plays a different role, but most are extremely important to human health. In addition, there are also microorganisms in the intestinal tract that can cause disease.

According to research, these gut microorganisms can weigh up to 2 - 5 pounds, equivalent to 1 - 2 kg (approximately the weight of a human brain). They combine with each other and act as an accessory organ in the body, playing a huge role in the overall health of a person.

How does the gut microbiota affect the body?

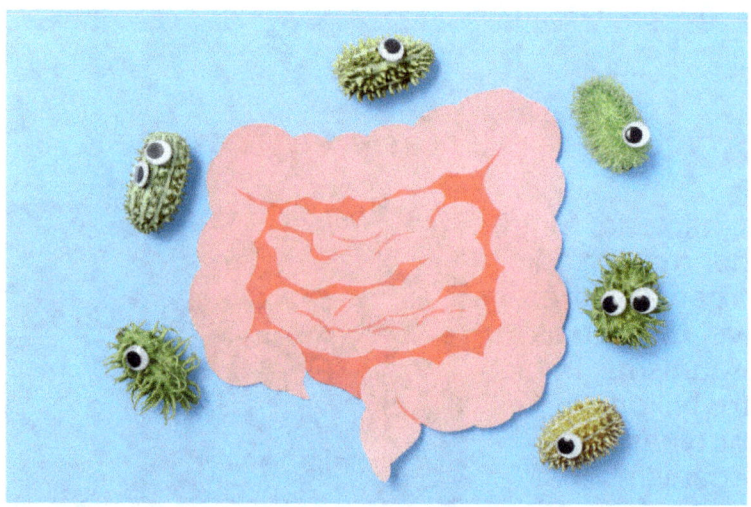

Humans have evolved to coexist with gut microorganisms for millions of years. Over the years, microorganisms in the gut have played many important roles in the human body. In fact, without the gut microbiome, it is very difficult for our bodies to survive.

Gut microbiota begins to affect the human body from the moment of birth. The first time a person comes into contact with the microorganism is when it passes through the mother's birth canal. However, some recent evidence shows that infants are exposed to certain types of microorganisms from the time they are in the womb.

As a child grows, the gut microbiome begins to become more diverse. The higher the diversity of your gut microbiome, the better for your health.

Interestingly, the foods that you consume every day have a significant effect on the diversity of your gut microbiota. As the microorganisms in the gut grow, they affect your body in a number of ways:

Digestion of breast milk: Some of the first bacteria begin to grow inside the infant's intestines organisms, also known collectively as Bifidobacteria. They digest the healthy sugars in breast milk - important for the development of babies.

Digesting fiber: Certain types of bacteria help digest fiber, producing short-chain fatty acids, which are important for gut health. Fiber can help prevent your body from developing diabetes, being overweight, heart disease, and cancer. Helps control the body's immune system: The gut microbiome is one of the important factors, helping to control the functioning of the immune system. By communicating with immune cells, the microorganisms in your gut can control how your body responds to infection. Helps control brain health: Many recent studies show that the gut microbiome also significantly affects the central nervous system - which controls brain functions.

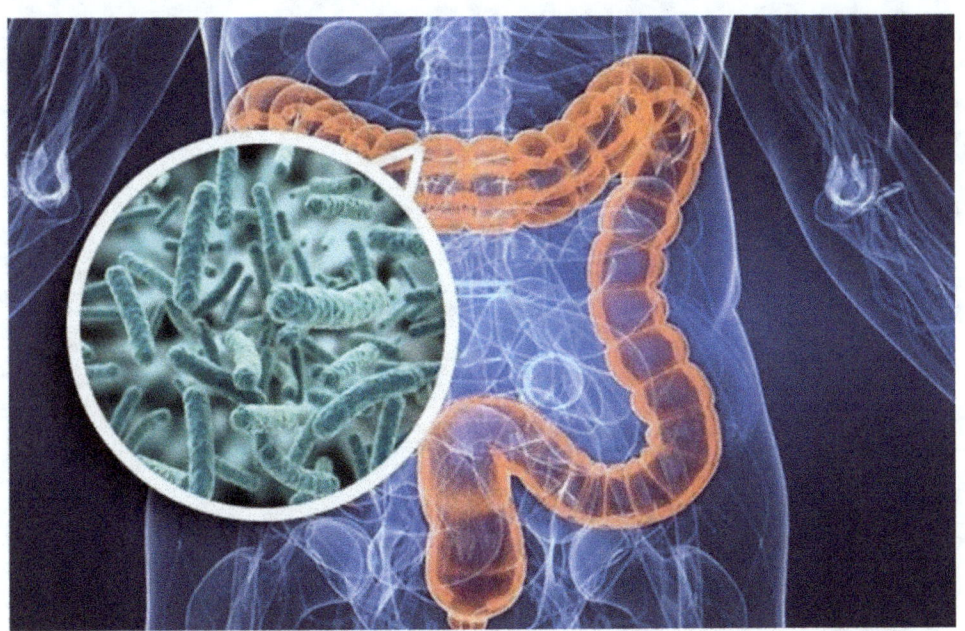

Gut microbiota affects body weight

In fact, there are thousands of different types of bacteria that live in your gut, and most of them are beneficial for your health. However, too much unhealthy bacteria in the gut can lead to illness.

An imbalance of beneficial microorganisms in the gut and unhealthy microorganisms is often referred to as a microbiome imbalance. This disorder can contribute to your weight gain, leading to weight gain.

Several studies have shown that the gut microbiome tends to be completely different between identical twins, one of whom is obese and the other very healthy. This demonstrates that differences in the gut microbiota are not genetic.

Nowadays, many people use probiotics because it is great for a healthy gut microbiome, and also helps support weight loss. However, the effect of probiotics on weight loss was relatively small (less than 1 kg of body weight was lost, the researchers said).

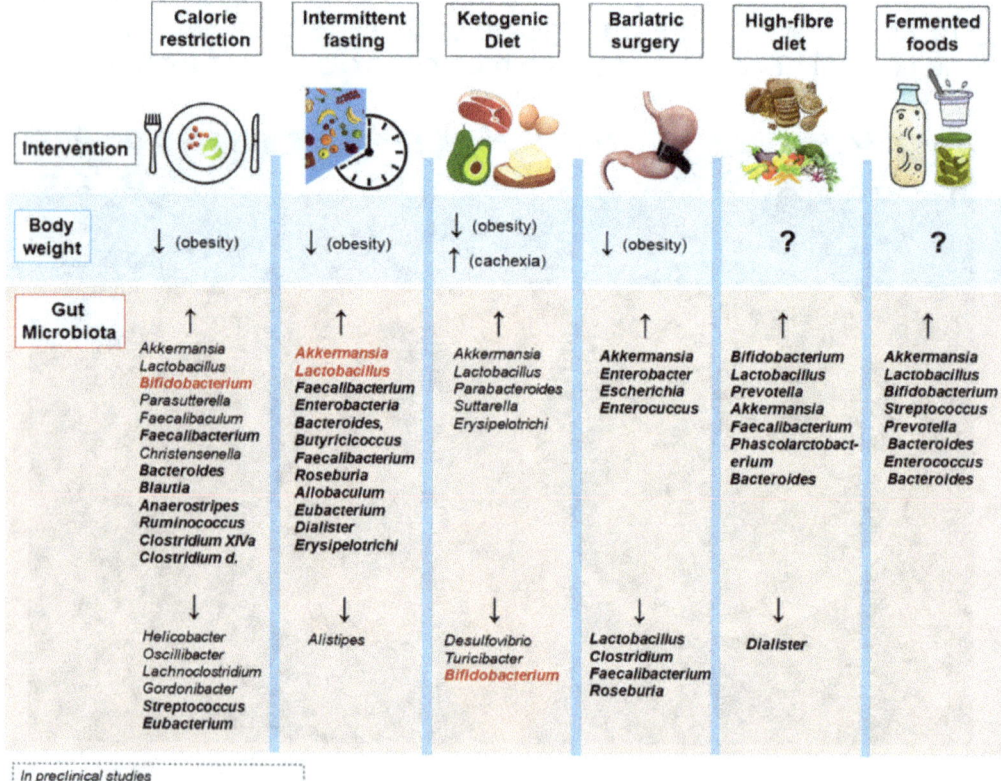

The gut microbiome has a big impact on gut health

The gut microbiome has a big influence on gut health. Many types of microorganisms are associated with intestinal problems, such as inflammatory bowel disease (IBD) and irritable bowel syndrome (IBS).
Symptoms such as bloating, abdominal pain, and cramping that people with IBS experience may be due to an imbalance in the microflora in the gut. These conditions are caused by intestinal bacteria that produce more gases and other chemicals, which contribute to unpleasant bowel symptoms.

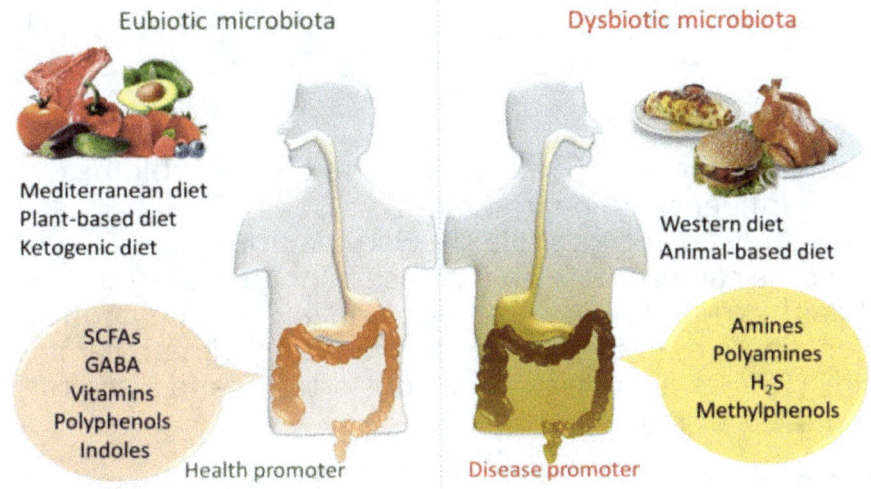

However, some beneficial microorganisms in the gut also help improve digestive system health. Probiotics like Lactobacilli and Bifidobacteria found in probiotics and yogurt have the ability to help seal the spaces between intestinal cells and prevent leaky gut syndrome (LGS).
In addition, these beneficial bacteria also help prevent disease-causing bacteria from attaching to the intestinal wall. In fact, taking certain probiotics containing Lactobacilli and Bifidobacteria can reduce the uncomfortable symptoms of IBS.

Gut microbiome benefits heart health

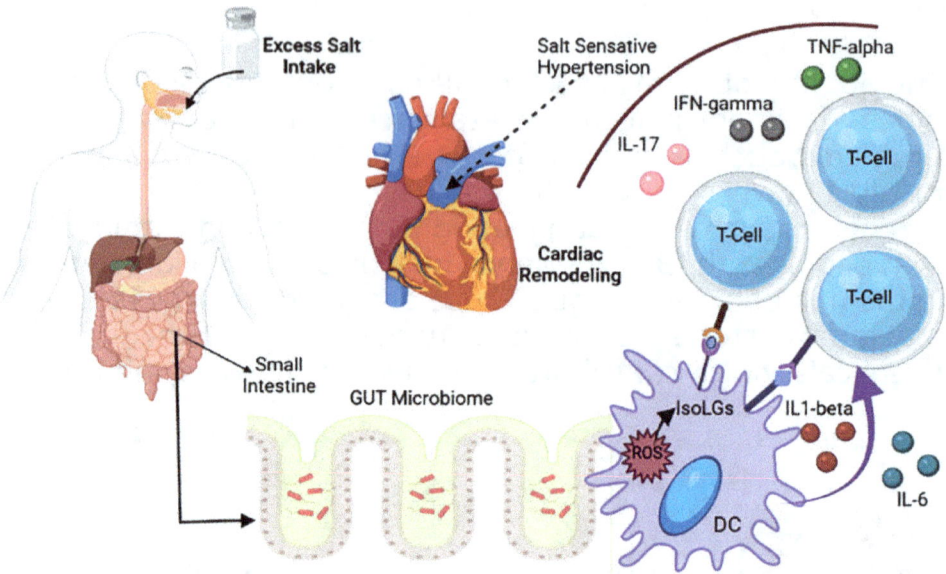

In addition to these important roles, the gut microbiome even has a big influence on heart health.
A recent study in 1500 people showed that the gut microbiome can promote an increase in good cholesterol HDL and healthy triglycerides. However, unhealthy gut microbes can contribute to heart disease by producing trimethylamine N-oxide (TMAO), a chemical that clogs arteries and leads to heart attacks or stroke.

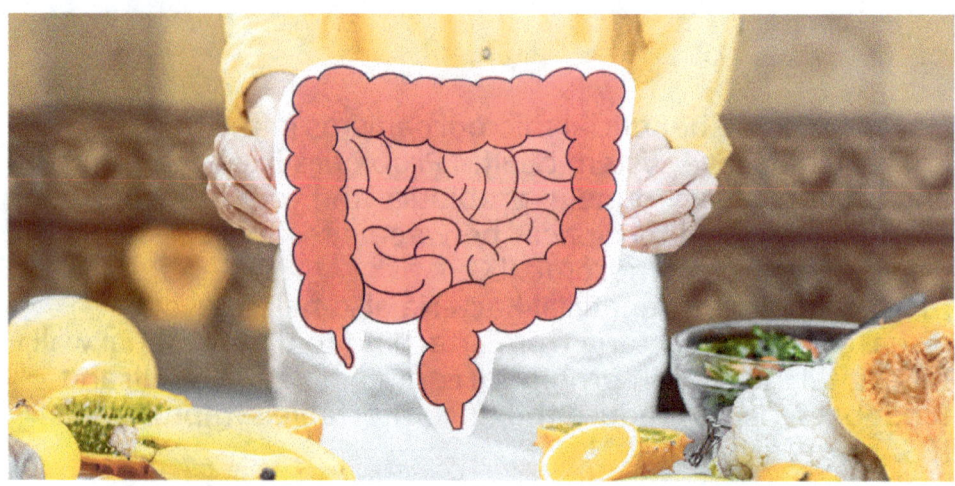

Some bacteria in the microbiome convert choline and L-carnitine into TMAO (both nutrients found in red meat and other animal food sources). This switch may increase risk factors for heart disease. However, other types of gut microbiota, particularly Lactobacilli, can help lower bad cholesterol levels when taken as probiotics.

Gut microbiota helps control blood sugar levels

Gut microbiota also help effectively control high blood sugar levels, which increase the risk of type 1 and type 2 diabetes. A recent study in 33 infants at high risk for diabetes Inherited type 1 diabetes has shown that the diversity of the gut microbiota is dramatically reduced before the onset of the disease. In addition, the experts also found that the levels of harmful gut microorganisms were increased just before the onset of type 1 diabetes in these children.
Some evidence also shows that, even when many people eat the same foods, their blood sugar levels can vary widely. This is due to the activity of microorganisms in the intestinal tract.

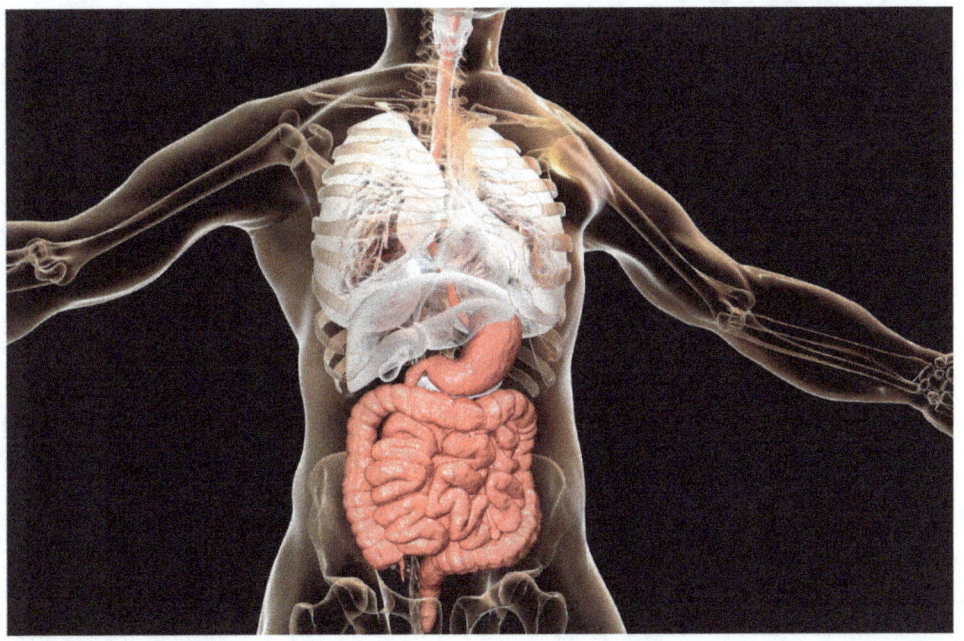

Gut microbiome affects brain health

Gut microbiota may even provide brain health benefits in a number of different ways.

Certain species of gut bacteria have the ability to produce brain chemicals called neurotransmitters. Typically the antidepressant neurotransmitter serotonin, is made mainly in the gut.

In fact, the human gut is physically connected to the brain through millions of nerves. Therefore, the gut microbiome may also influence brain health by controlling the messages sent to the brain by these nerves.

Experts say that people with different psychological disorders often have different species of microorganisms in the gut than healthy people. This demonstrates that the gut microbiome has a major influence on brain health.

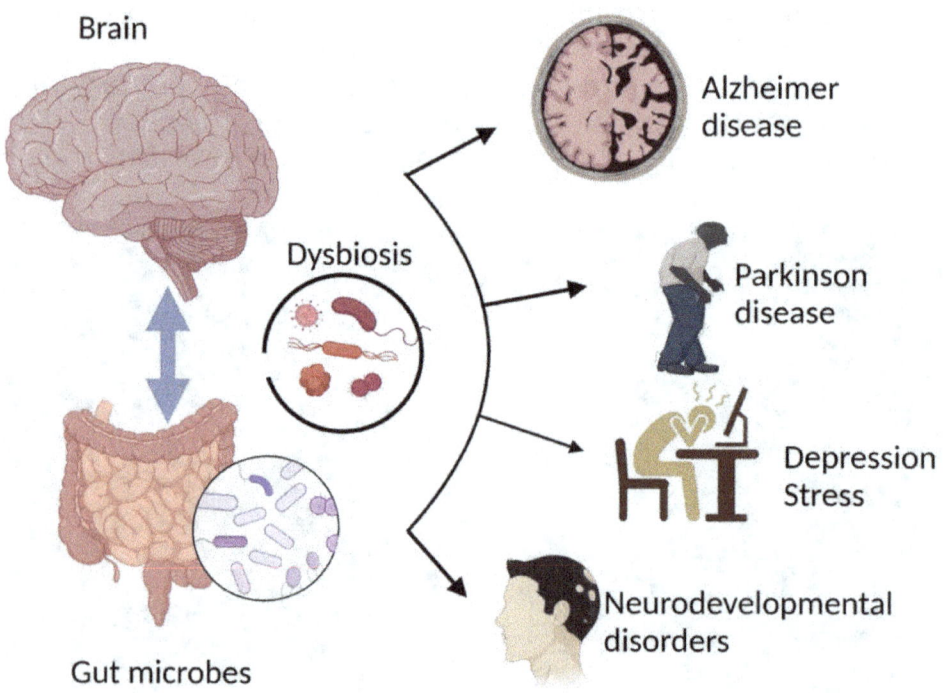

EXERCISES THAT SUPPORT GUT HEALTH

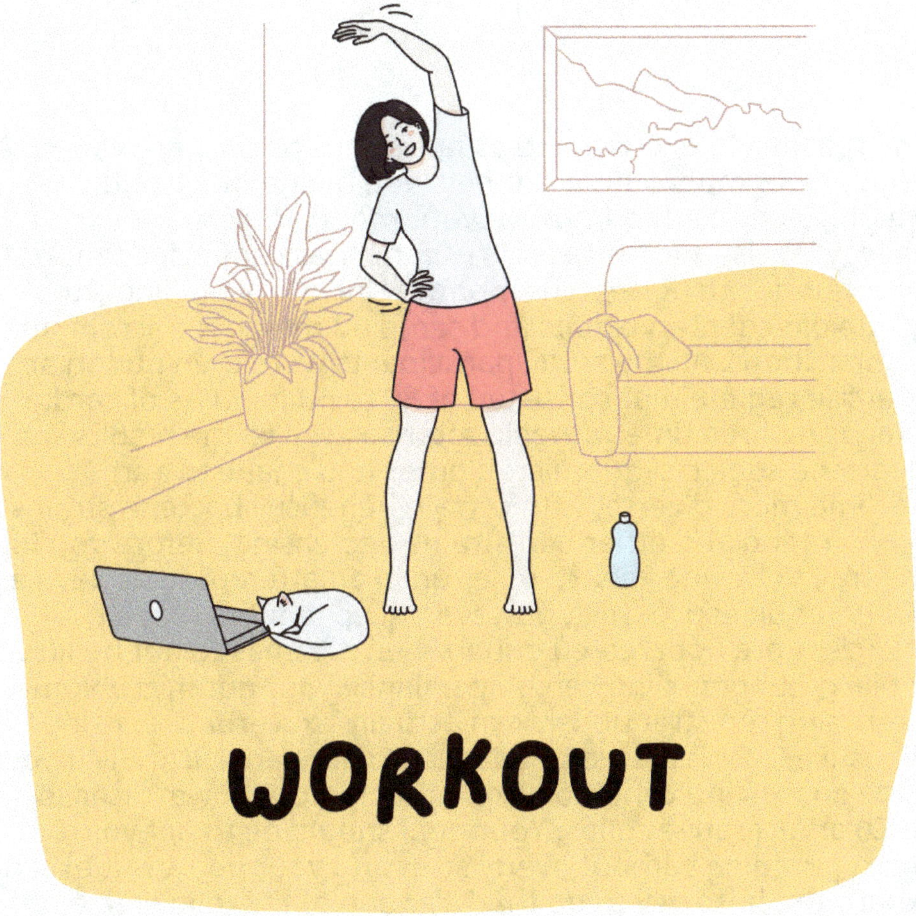

WORKOUT

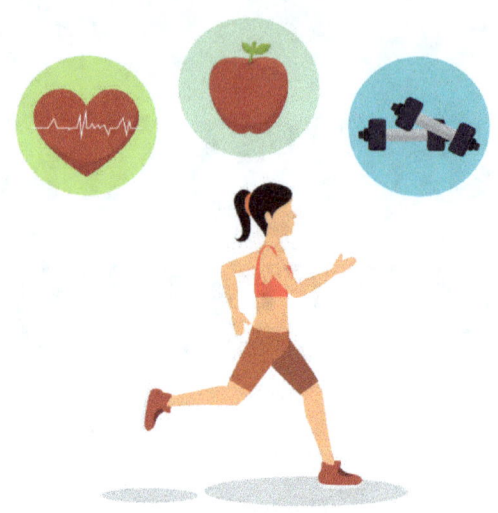

The reasons to exercise are as numerous as they are varied. A regular workout routine can help you maintain a healthy weight, sleep better, improve your mood, increase your energy levels--and, as recent research has confirmed, improve your gut health. Researchers at the University of Illinois took a group of sedentary adults and sampled their gut microbiome compositions. All the study participants were then put on an exercise regime that consisted of 30 to 60 minutes of cardio exercises three times a week. After six weeks, the results were clear: the subjects' gut microbiomes had changed and become more diverse, with certain beneficial bacteria strains proliferating and other bad strains decreasing. Before you hit the trail for a vigorous 10-mile run in an attempt to achieve a healthier digestive tract, however, keep in mind that all exercises are not created equal when it comes to gut health. While getting moving can help balance your gut microbiome, exercising too strenuously can actually exacerbate existing digestive tract issues such as inflammation, particularly if you have an existing condition like inflammatory bowel disease (IBD) or ulcerative colitis. Your goal should be to get your heart pumping without overly stressing your body. But exactly what's the best way to do that? Try one of the following eight low-impact (yet highly effective!) exercises--and remember to continue to support your gut health efforts by eating healthy, drinking plenty of water, and taking a daily probiotic supplement.

YOGA

Yoga has a well-earned reputation for helping people slim down, tone up and get healthier while being gentle on the body, making it an excellent option for those looking to reduce stress and improve gut health. What's more, there's a significant body of research to back up yoga's particular benefits for digestive health. One study found that those with inflammatory bowel disease experienced fewer symptoms when following an exercise regime that included an hour of yoga a day. Additional research has shown that the gut health promoting effects of yoga work equally well for children and adolescents with irritable bowel syndrome. In other words, spring for a group package at the local yoga studio, as the entire family can benefit from taking a yoga class or two!

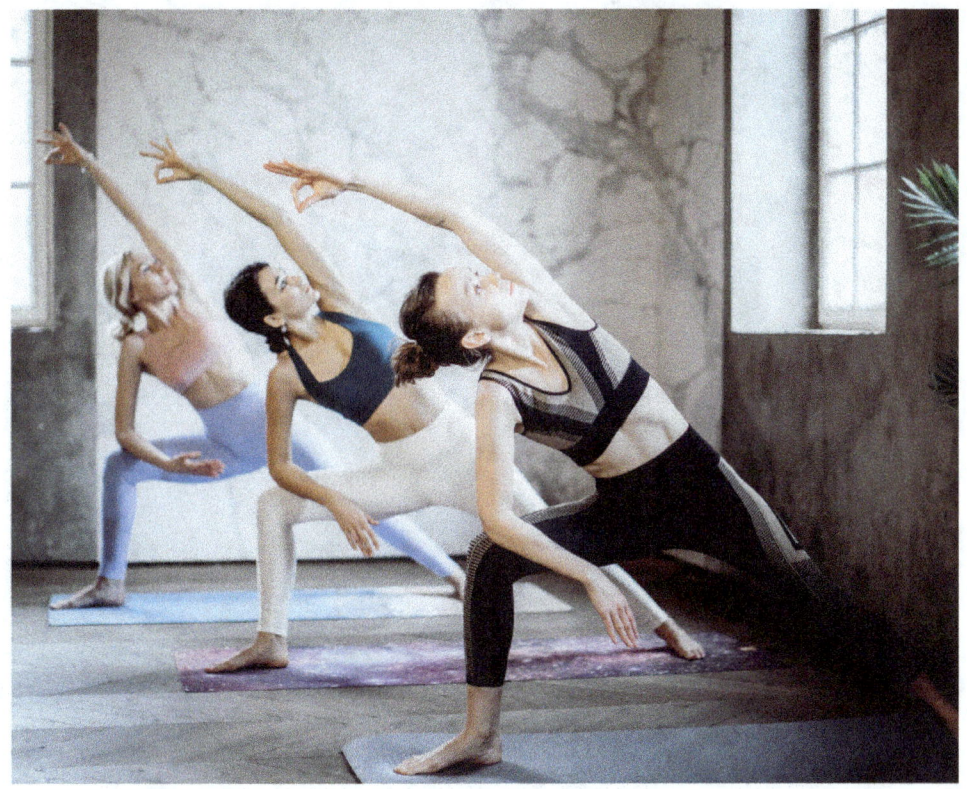

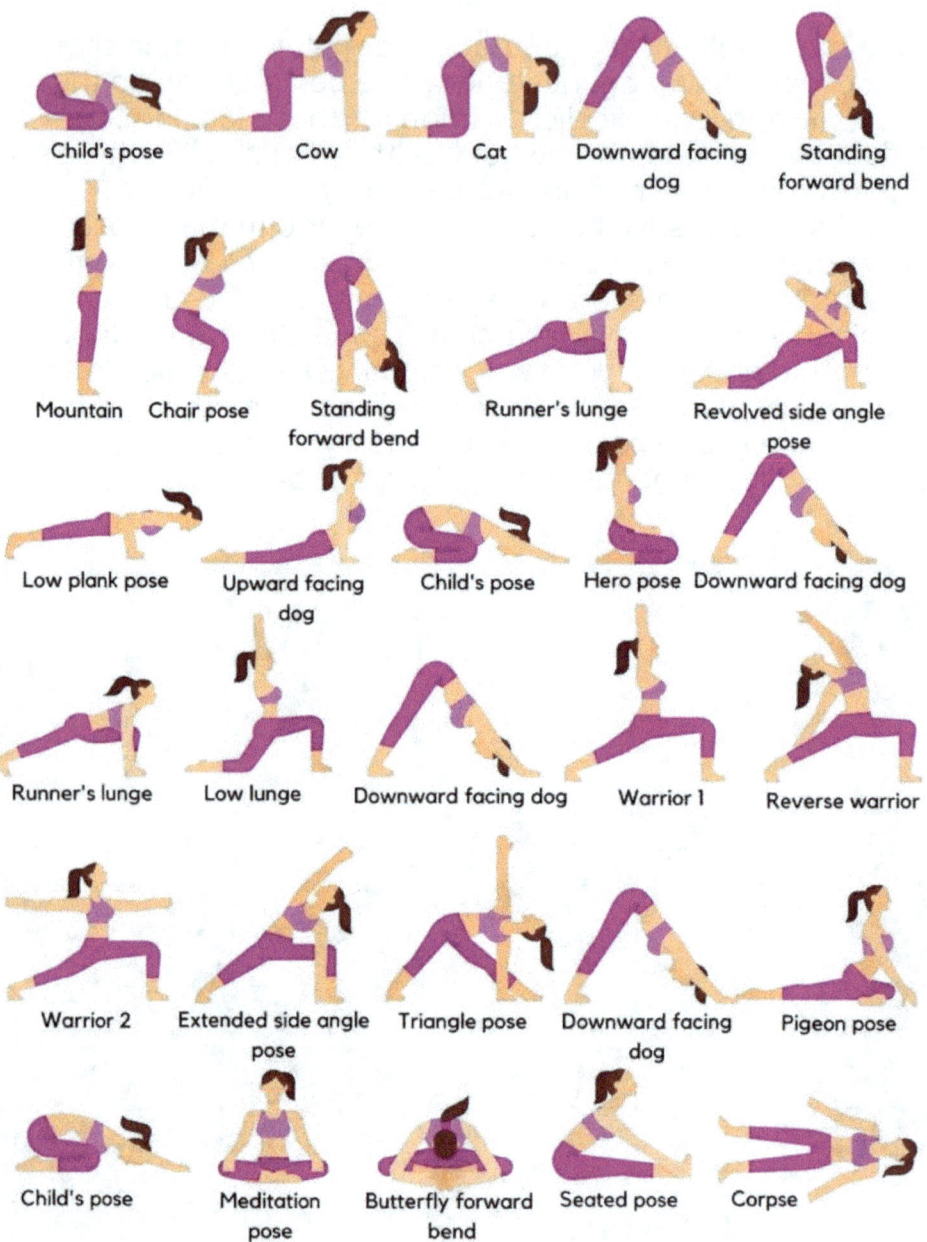

JOGGING

One of the exercises that the University of Illinois' study participants could choose was jogging--and as the results of that study show, jogging is an excellent choice for those looking to bolster the diversity of their gut microbiome.

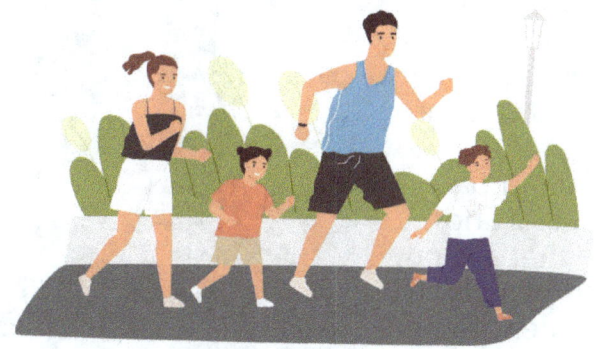

 Whether indoors on a treadmill or outside on a trail, a steady jog can dramatically improve your health. The key (as with all exercises on this list) is to work hard enough to break a sweat but not so hard that you overstress your body.

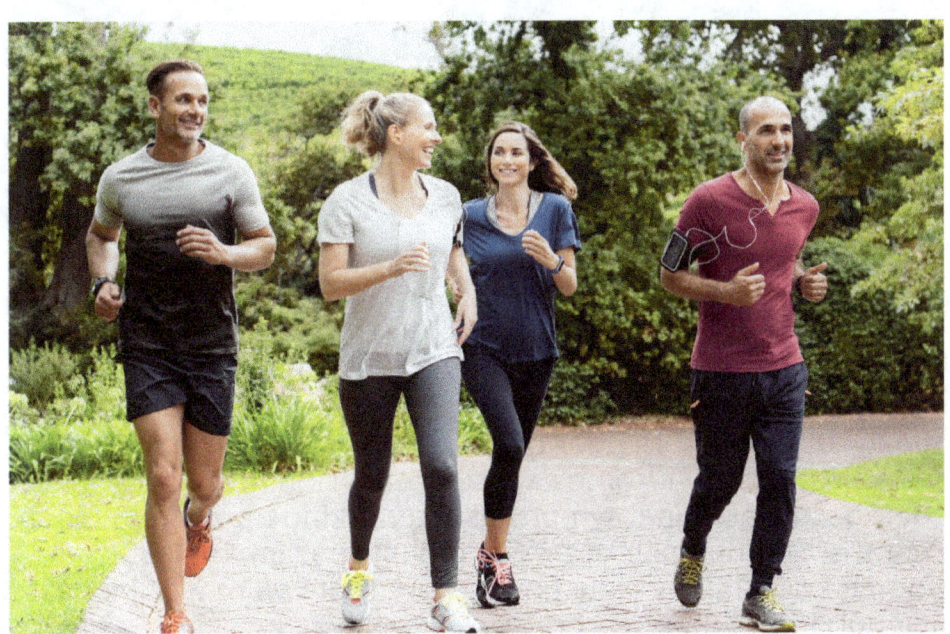

WALKING

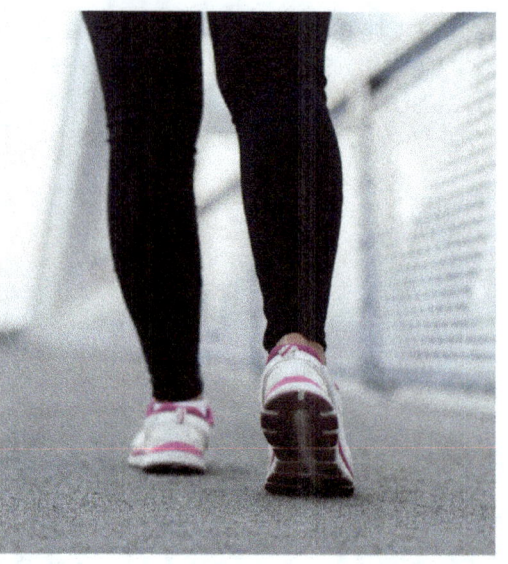

It can be easy to dismiss walking as an effective exercise routine. In the age of high-intensity workouts, walking just doesn't seem painful enough to work. In actually, walking is one of the best exercises you can do:
it's extremely low-impact, it's an excellent starting point for those that are new to exercise, and you don't need any equipment to get started.

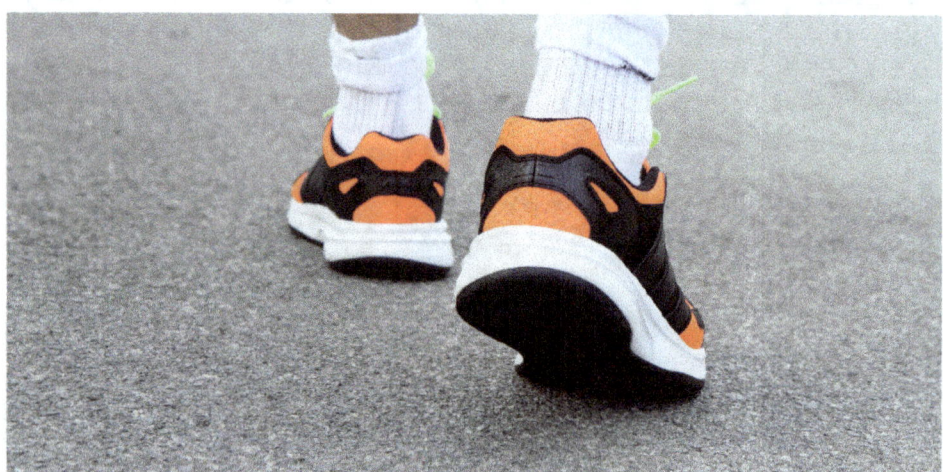

 As with yoga, walking has been shown in studies to help those suffering from poor gut health; study participants with irritable bowel syndrome experienced a significant drop in their gastrointestinal symptoms after taking up walking for six months. So put a pair of comfortable shoes on and get yourself out the door--just make sure that you're walking fast enough to get that heart rate up

SWIMMING

Perhaps the ultimate in low-impact exercises, swimming is a particularly good choice for those who want to improve gut health while also protecting joint health.

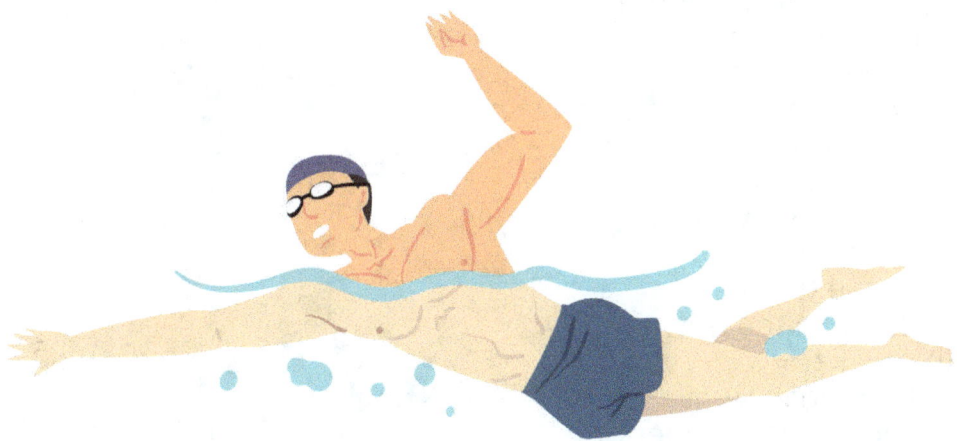

One caveat here: spending too much time in heavily-chlorinated pools (like most public pools are) can be counterproductive in terms of gut health, as the high levels of chlorine may have an effect on the good bacteria in your gut as well as the bad bacteria that can grow in pools. To the extent possible, trying swimming in fresh water. Hey, it's the perfect excuse for a trip to the beach!

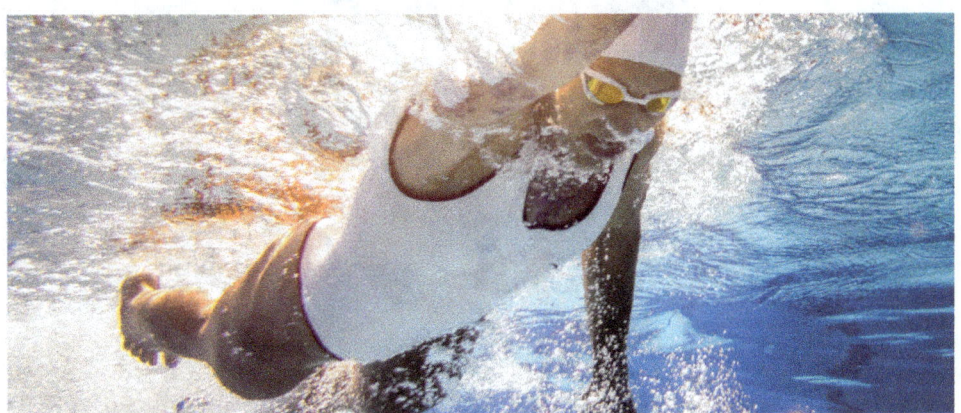

CYCLING

On the road or in the gym, cycling is another great option for digestive health. Research has shown that low- to moderate-intensity cycling done for approximately three hours a week can increase the good bacteria in the gut (particularly Akkermansia) while lowering the number of bad strains (such as Proteobacteria).

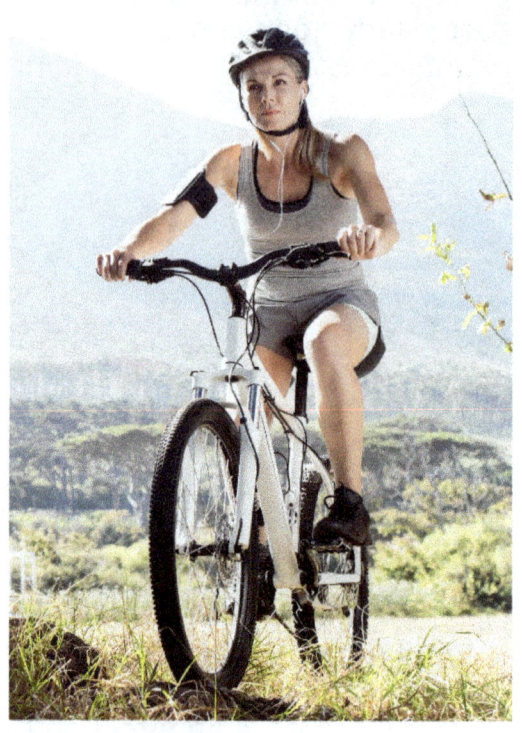

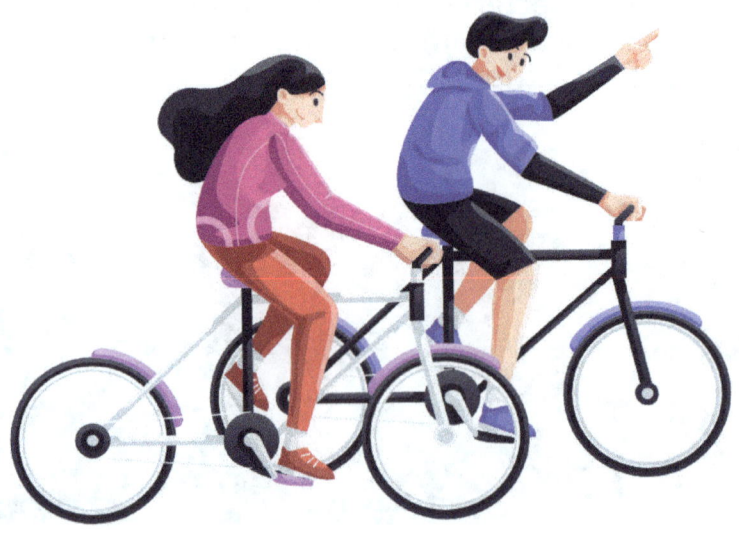

ELLIPTICAL

Like walking, jogging, and cycling, using the elliptical machine was one of the options offered to the University of Illinois' study participants, proving its effectiveness at promoting gut health. The biggest benefit of using an elliptical machine over the other three exercises is that it lowers the amount of weight that the lower body must bear, making it better for those with chronic lower-body injuries.

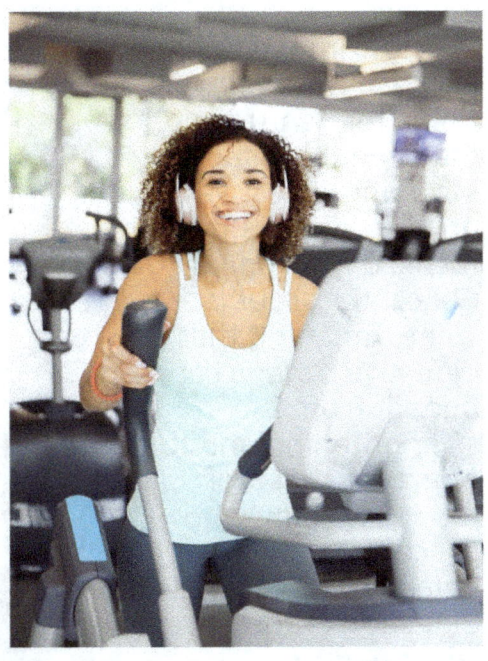

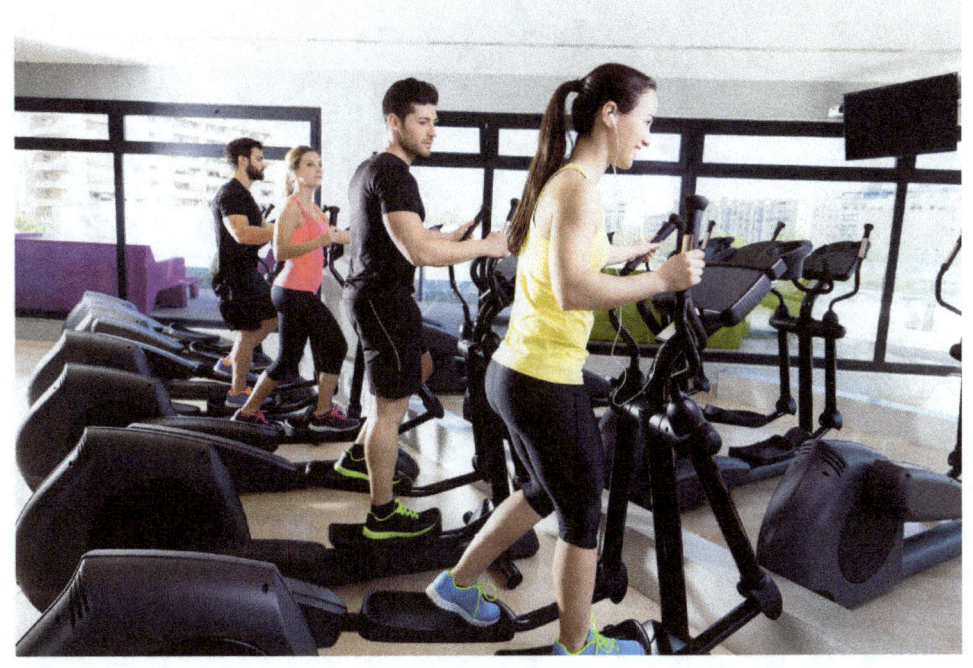

TAI CHI

This low-impact, gentle exercise has been used in China for centuries to treat many health issues, including digestive tract problems. The slow and focused movements of Tai Chi center around the spine, meaning that the digestive organs can also benefit from the strengthening and toning effects of these circular motions. Many who practice Tai Chi note that it helps promote regular digestion and relieve constipation.

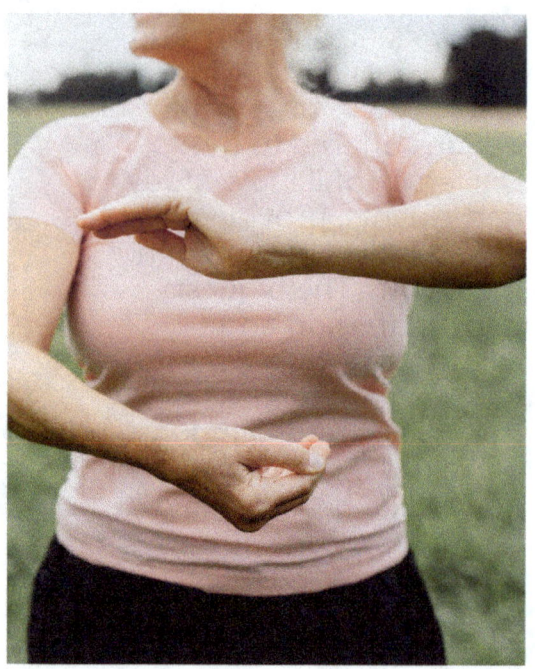

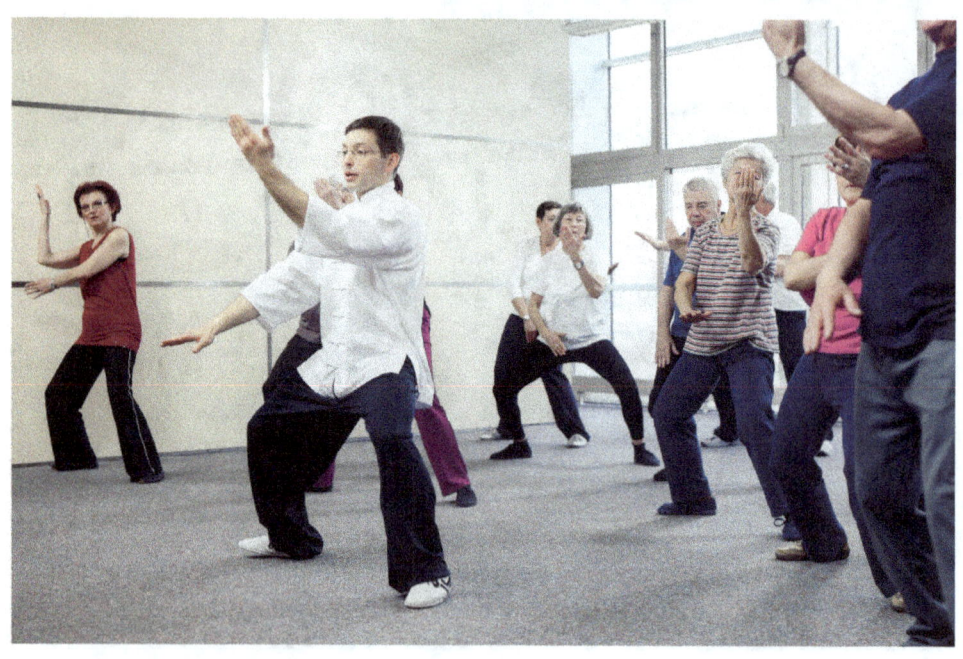

PILATES

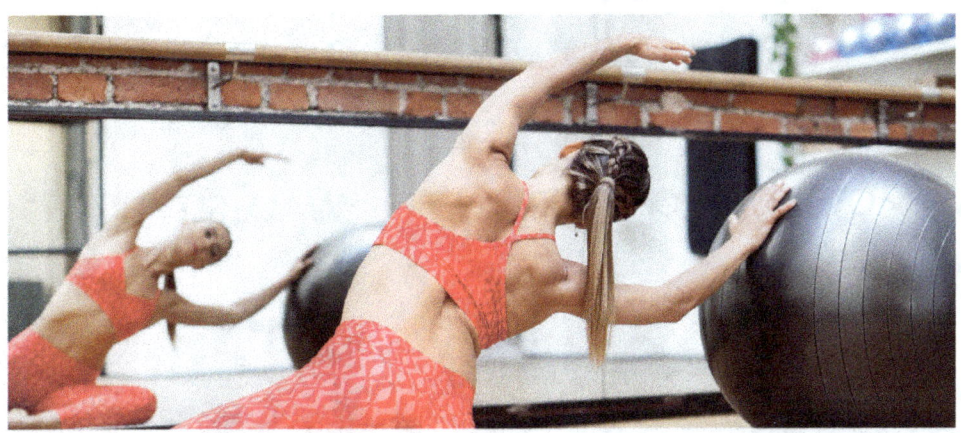

Similar to yoga, Pilates focuses on balance, posture, and flexibility, making it an excellent low-stress workout option. As an added bonus, several common Pilates moves--such as cat-cow and articulated bridge--work the muscles of the deep core in such a way as to promote proper digestion.

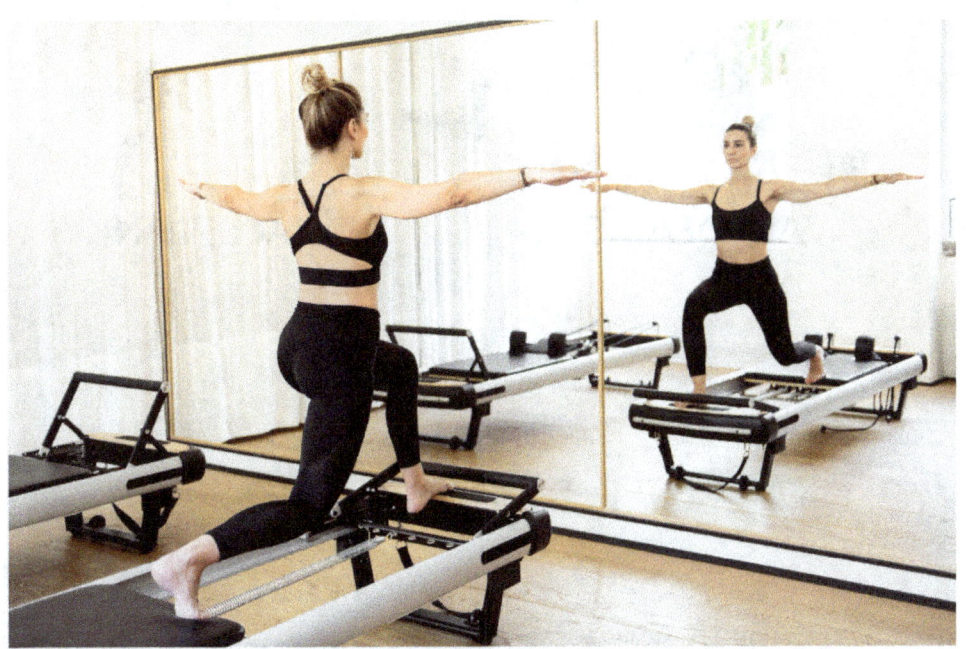

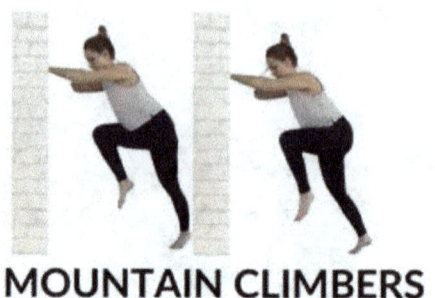
MOUNTAIN CLIMBERS

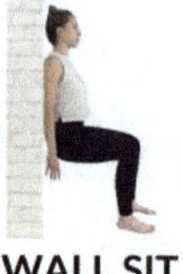
WALL SIT

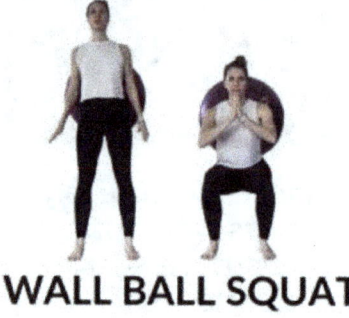
WALL BALL SQUAT

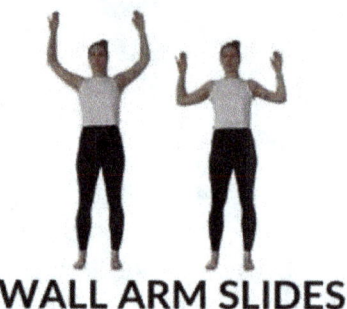
WALL ARM SLIDES

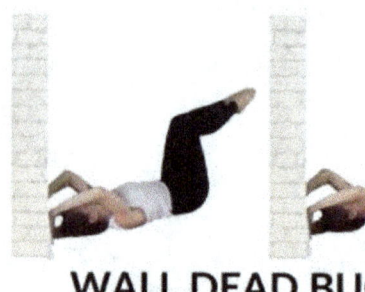
WALL DEAD BUG

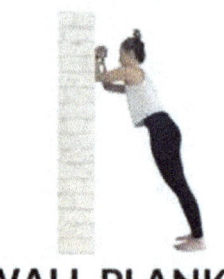
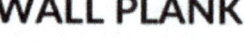
WALL PLANK

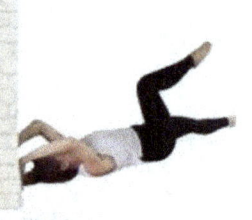
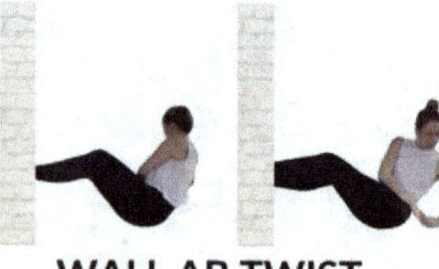
WALL AB TWIST

CHOOSE YOUR EXERCISE PLAN

Keep in mind that the particular exercise routine that you choose is less important than choosing one that you can keep up. Remember the University of Illinois study that we talked about above? After embarking on a workout routine for six weeks and seeing their gut health improve, participants were directed to return to their sedentary lifestyle for another six weeks. Perhaps unsurprisingly, their gut microbiomes also returned to their previous unbalanced, unhealthy state.

The conclusion here is clear: exercise needs to be a regular habit to truly affect any meaningful change in your gut health. So lace up your sneakers, hit the gym!

30 DAY Fitness CHALLENGE

MONDAY	TUESDAY	WEDNESDAY	THURSDAY	FRIDAY	SATURDAY	SUNDAY
Day 1	Day 2	Day 3	Day 4	Day 5	Day 6	Day 7
Day 8	Day 9	Day 10	Day 11	Day 12	Day 13	Day 14
Day 15	Day 16	Day 17	Day 18	Day 19	Day 20	Day 21
Day 22	Day 23	Day 24	Day 25	Day 26	Day 27	Day 28
Day 29	Day 30	believe in yourself	you are worth it	one day closer	think long term	keep going

TIPS FOR HEALTHY EATING

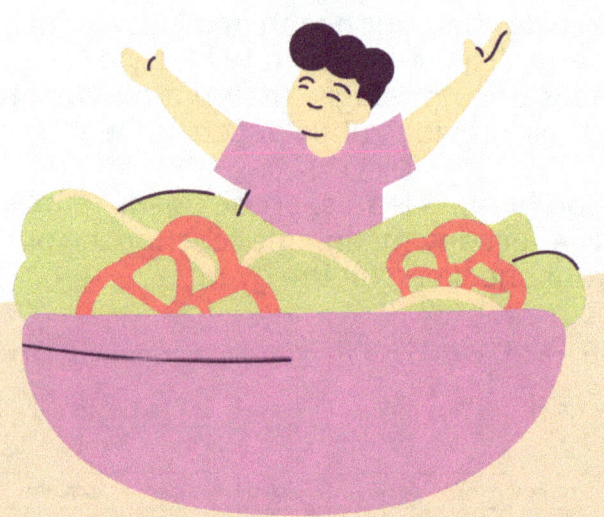

MAINTAIN A HEALTHY DIET

These practical tips cover the basics of healthy eating and can help you make healthier choices.

The key to a healthy diet is to eat the right amount of calories for how active you are so you balance the energy you consume with the energy you use.

If you eat or drink more than your body needs, you'll put on weight because the energy you do not use is stored as fat. If you eat and drink too little, you'll lose weight.

You should also eat a wide range of foods to make sure you're getting a balanced diet and your body is receiving all the nutrients it needs.

It's recommended that men have around 2,500 calories a day (10,500 kilojoules). Women should have around 2,000 calories a day (8,400 kilojoules).

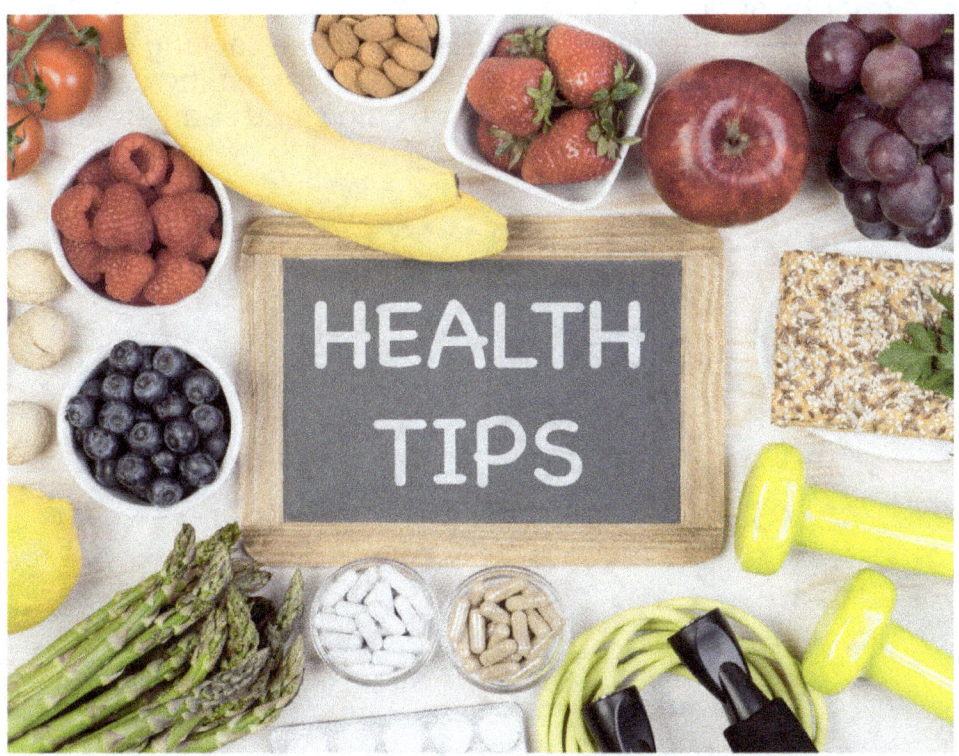

BASE YOUR MEALS ON HIGHER FIBRE STARCHY CARBOHYDRATES

Starchy carbohydrates should make up just over a third of the food you eat. They include potatoes, bread, rice, pasta and cereals.
Choose higher fibre or wholegrain varieties, such as wholewheat pasta, brown rice or potatoes with their skins on. They contain more fibre than white or refined starchy carbohydrates and can help you feel full for longer.
Try to include at least 1 starchy food with each main meal. Some people think starchy foods are fattening, but gram for gram the carbohydrate they contain provides fewer than half the calories of fat.
Keep an eye on the fats you add when you're cooking or serving these types of foods because that's what increases the calorie content – for example, oil on chips, butter on bread and creamy sauces on pasta.

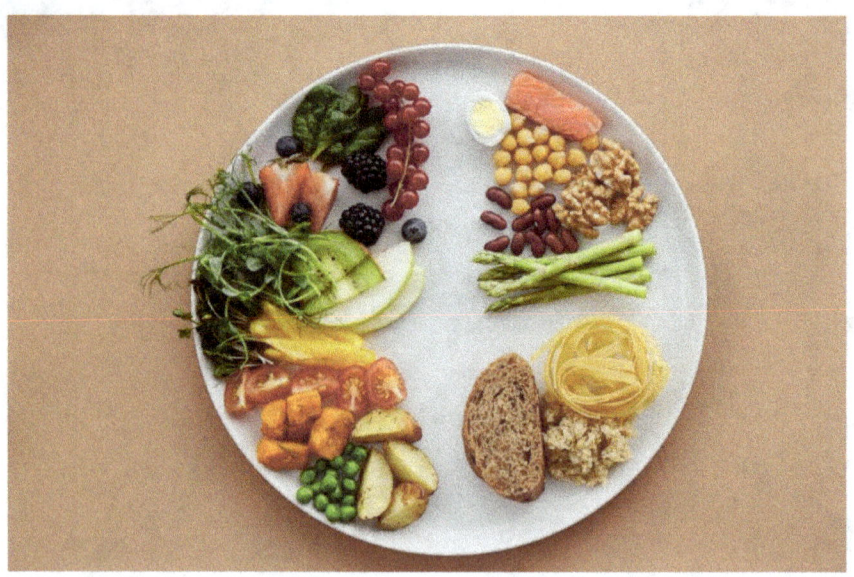

Tips for eating more starchy foods

These tips can help you increase the amount of starchy foods in your diet.

Breakfast
- Choose wholegrain cereals, or mix some in with your favourite healthy breakfast cereals.
- Plain porridge with fruit makes a warming winter breakfast.
- Whole oats with fruit and low-fat, lower-sugar yoghurt makes a tasty summer breakfast.

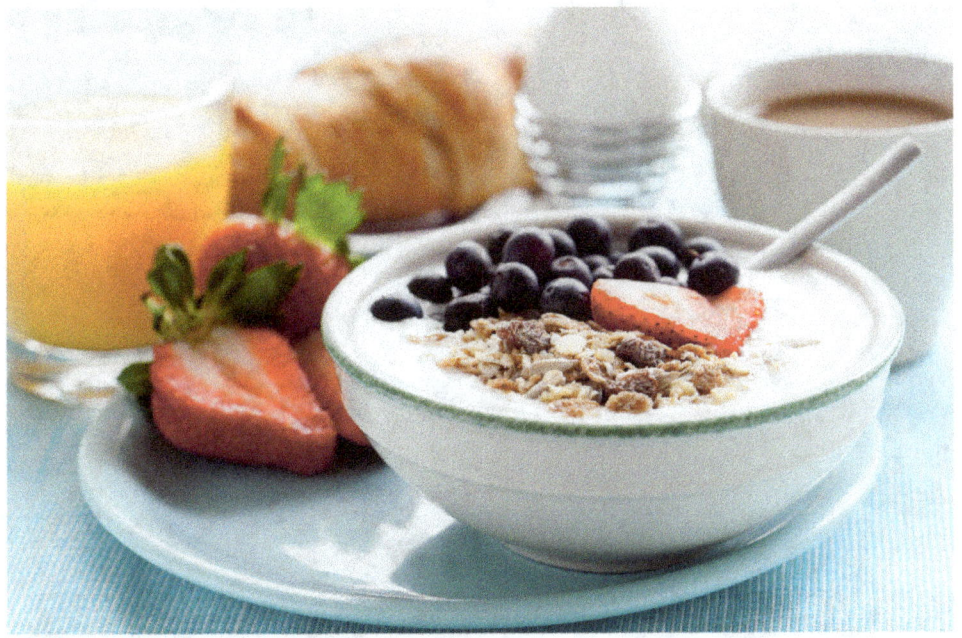

Lunch and dinner
- Try a baked potato for lunch – eat the skin for even more fibre.
- Instead of having chips or frying potatoes, try making oven-baked potato wedges.
- Have more rice or pasta and less sauce – but do not skip the vegetables.

- Try breads such as seeded, wholemeal or granary. When you choose wholegrain varieties, you'll also increase the amount of fibre you're eating.
- Try brown rice – it makes a very tasty rice salad.

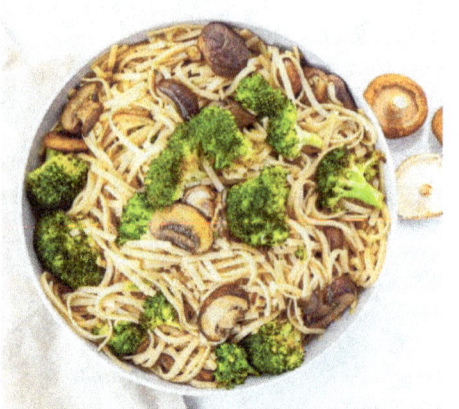

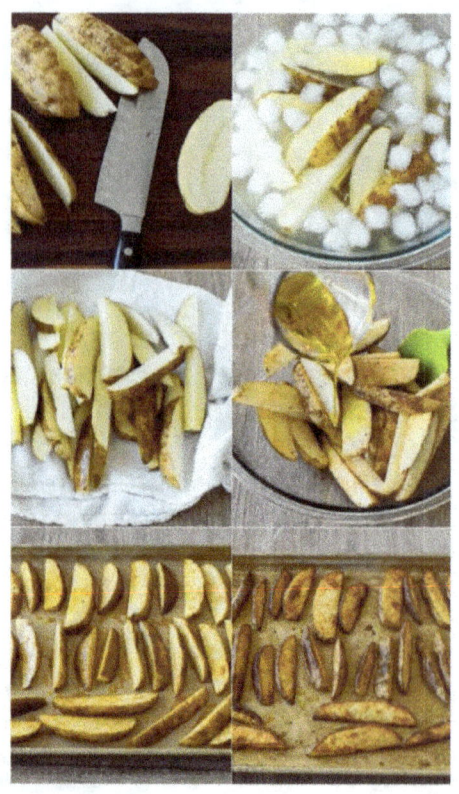

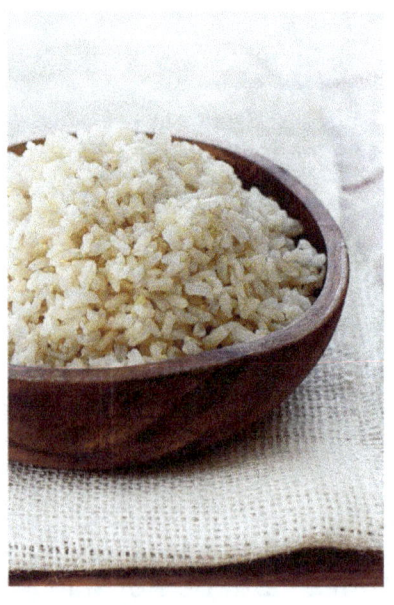

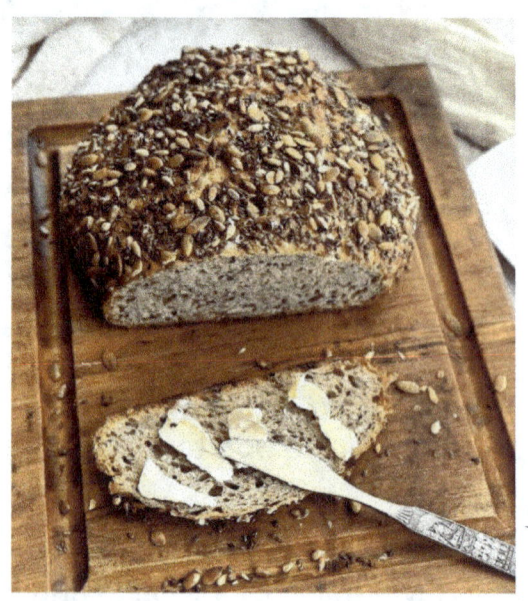

Types of starchy foods

- **Potatoes**

Potatoes are a great choice of starchy food and a good source of energy, fibre, B vitamins and potassium.
In the UK, we also get a lot of our vitamin C from potatoes. Although potatoes only contain a small amount of vitamin C, we generally eat a lot of them. They're good value for money and can be a healthy choice.
Although potatoes are a vegetable, in the UK we mostly eat them as the starchy food part of a meal, and they're a good source of carbohydrate in our diet.

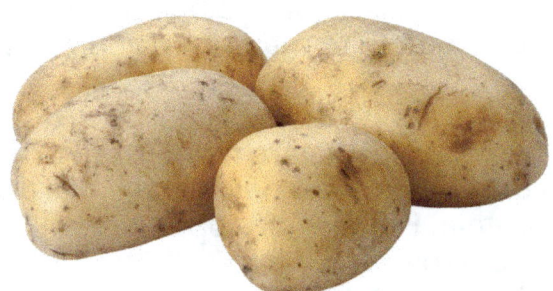

- **Bread**

Bread, especially wholemeal, granary, brown and seeded varieties, is a healthy choice to eat as part of a balanced diet. Wholegrain, wholemeal and brown breads give us energy and contain B vitamins, vitamin E, fibre and a wide range of minerals.
White bread also contains a range of vitamins and minerals, but it has less fibre than wholegrain, wholemeal or brown bread.

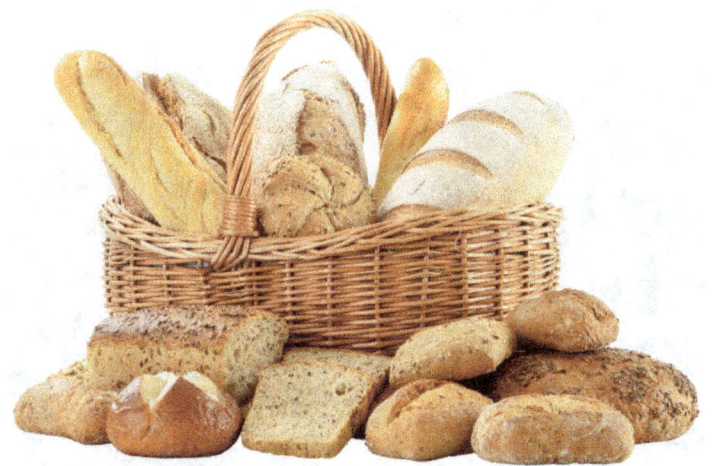

If you prefer white bread, look for higher-fibre options.
Some people avoid bread because they're concerned about having a food intolerance or allergy to wheat, or they think bread is fattening.
However, completely cutting out any type of food from your diet could mean you miss out on a range of nutrients that you need to stay healthy.
If you're concerned that you have a wheat allergy or intolerance, speak to a GP.
Bread can be stored at room temperature. Follow the "best before" date to make sure you eat it fresh.

- **Cereal products**

Cereal products are made from grains. Wholegrain cereals can contribute to our daily intake of iron, fibre, B vitamins and protein. Higher-fibre options can also provide a slow release of energy.
Wheat, oats, barley, rye and rice are commonly available cereals that can be eaten as wholegrains.
This means cereal products consisting of oats or oatmeal, such as porridge, and wholewheat products are healthy breakfast options.
Barley, couscous, corn and tapioca also count as healthy cereal products.
Many cereal products in the UK are refined, with low wholegrain content. They can also be high in added salt and sugar.
When you're shopping for cereals, check the food labels to compare different products.

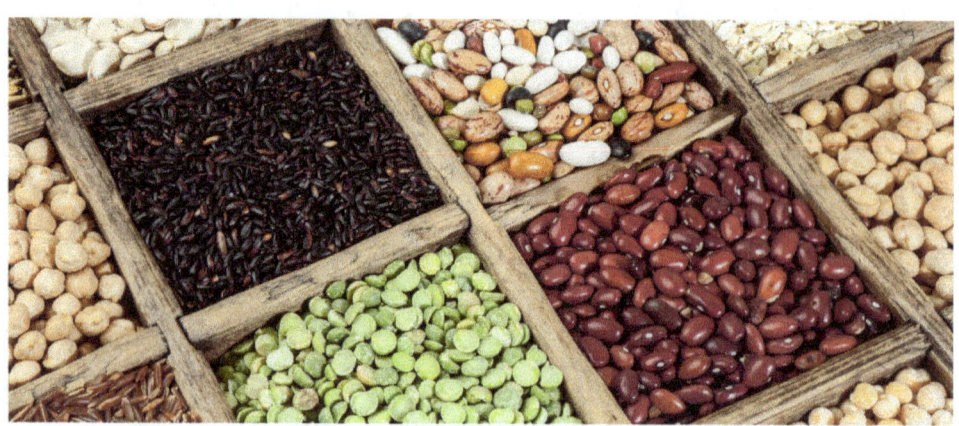

- **Rice and grains**

Rice and grains are an excellent choice of starchy food. They give us energy, are low in fat, and good value for money.

There are many types to choose from, including:
-all kinds of rice – such as quick-cook, arborio, basmati, long grain, brown, short grain and wild
-couscous
-bulgur wheat

As well as carbohydrates, rice and grains (particularly brown and wholegrain varieties) can contain:

-fibre, which can help your body get rid of waste products
-B vitamins, which help release energy from the food you eat and help your body work properly

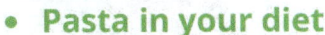

Rice and grains, such as couscous and bulgur wheat, can be eaten hot or cold, and in salads.

- **Pasta in your diet**

Pasta is another healthy option to base your meal on. It consists of dough made from durum wheat and water and contains iron and B vitamins.

Wholewheat or wholegrain are healthier than ordinary pasta, as they contain more fibre. We digest wholegrain foods slower than refined grains, so they can help us feel full for longer.

Dried pasta can be stored in a cupboard and typically has a long shelf life, while fresh pasta will need to be refrigerated and has a shorter lifespan.

Check the food packaging for "best before" or "use by" dates and further storage instructions.

EAT LOTS OF FRUIT AND VEG

It's recommended that you eat at least 5 portions of a variety of fruit and veg every day. They can be fresh, frozen, canned, dried or juiced.
Getting your 5 A Day is easier than it sounds. Why not chop a banana over your breakfast cereal, or swap your usual mid-morning snack for a piece of fresh fruit?
A portion of fresh, canned or frozen fruit and vegetables is 80g. A portion of dried fruit (which should be kept to mealtimes) is 30g.
A 150ml glass of fruit juice, vegetable juice or smoothie also counts as 1 portion, but limit the amount you have to no more than 1 glass a day as these drinks are sugary and can damage your teeth.

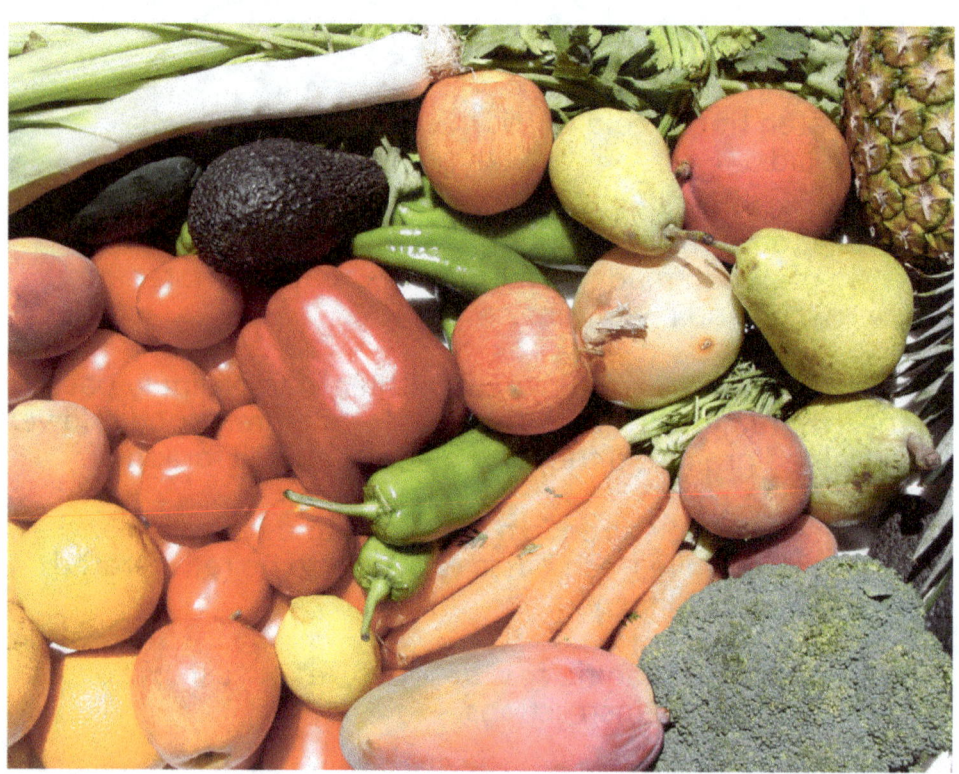

EAT MORE FISH, INCLUDING A PORTION OF OILY FISH

Fish is a good source of protein and contains many vitamins and minerals.
Aim to eat at least 2 portions of fish a week, including at least 1 portion of oily fish.
Oily fish are high in omega-3 fats, which may help prevent heart disease.
Oily fish include:
- salmon
- trout
- herring
- sardines
- pilchards
- mackerel

Non-oily fish include:
- haddock
- plaice
- coley
- cod
- tuna
- skate
- hake

You can choose from fresh, frozen and canned, but remember that canned and smoked fish can be high in salt.

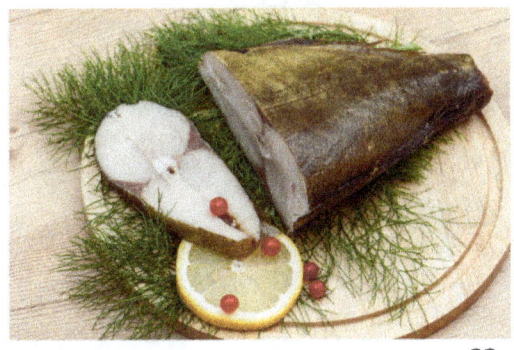
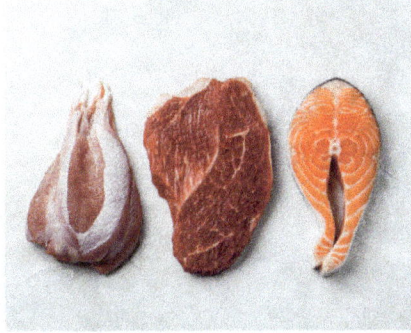

CUT DOWN ON SATURATED FAT AND SUGAR

Saturated fat

You need some fat in your diet, but it's important to pay attention to the amount and type of fat you're eating.
There are 2 main types of fat: saturated and unsaturated. Too much saturated fat can increase the amount of cholesterol in the blood, which increases your risk of developing heart disease.
On average, men should have no more than 30g of saturated fat a day. On average, women should have no more than 20g of saturated fat a day.
Children under the age of 11 should have less saturated fat than adults, but a low-fat diet is not suitable for children under 5. In addition, full-fat dairy products, such as cheese, fromage frais and yoghurt, are recommended up to the age of 2 years.
Saturated fat is found in many foods, such as:
- fatty cuts of meat
- sausages
- butter
- hard cheese
- cream
- cakes
- biscuits
- lard
- pies

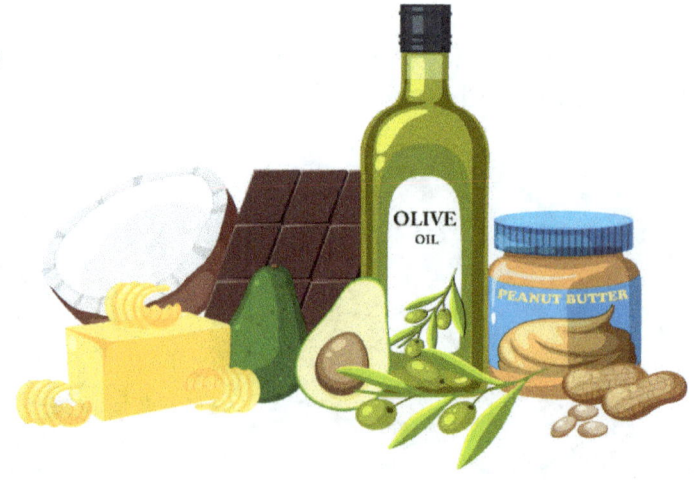

Try to eat less saturated fat and choose foods that contain unsaturated fats instead, such as vegetable oils and spreads, oily fish and avocados.
For a healthier choice, use a small amount of vegetable or olive oil, or reduced-fat spread instead of butter, lard or ghee.
When you're having meat, choose lean cuts and cut off any visible fat.
All types of fat are high in energy, so they should only be eaten in small amounts.

Sugar

Regularly consuming foods and drinks high in sugar increases your risk of obesity and tooth decay.
Sugary foods and drinks are often high in energy (measured in kilojoules or calories), and if consumed too often can contribute to weight gain. They can also cause tooth decay, especially if eaten between meals.
Free sugars are any sugars added to foods or drinks, or found naturally in honey, syrups and unsweetened fruit juices and smoothies.
This is the type of sugar you should be cutting down on, rather than the sugar found in fruit and milk.
Many packaged foods and drinks contain surprisingly high amounts of free sugars.

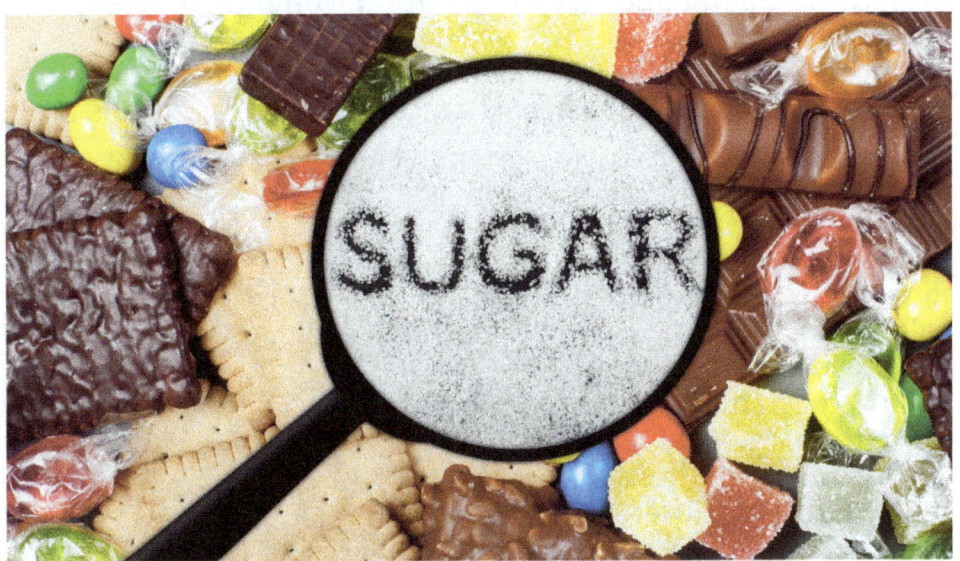

Free sugars are found in many foods, such as:
- sugary fizzy drinks
- sugary breakfast cereals
- cakes
- biscuits
- pastries and puddings
- sweets and chocolate
- alcoholic drinks

Food labels can help. Use them to check how much sugar foods contain.

More than 22.5g of total sugars per 100g means the food is high in sugar, while 5g of total sugars or less per 100g means the food is low in sugar.

EAT LESS SALT: NO MORE THAN 6G A DAY FOR ADULTS

Eating too much salt can raise your blood pressure. People with high blood pressure are more likely to develop heart disease or have a stroke.

Even if you do not add salt to your food, you may still be eating too much.

About three-quarters of the salt you eat is already in the food when you buy it, such as breakfast cereals, soups, breads and sauces.

Use food labels to help you cut down. More than 1.5g of salt per 100g means the food is high in salt.

Adults and children aged 11 and over should eat no more than 6g of salt (about a teaspoonful) a day. Younger children should have even less.

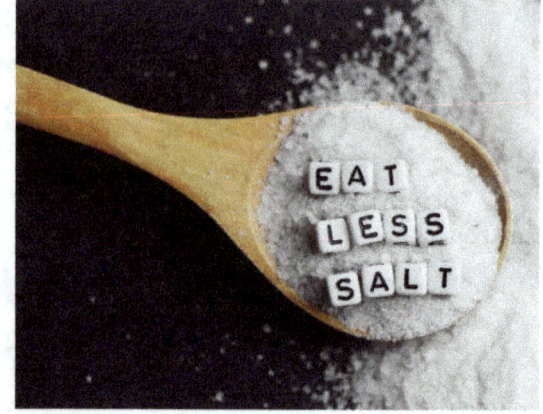

GET ACTIVE AND BE A HEALTHY WEIGHT

As well as eating healthily, regular exercise may help reduce your risk of getting serious health conditions. It's also important for your overall health and wellbeing.

Read more about the benefits of exercise and physical activity guidelines for adults.

Being overweight or obese can lead to health conditions, such as type 2 diabetes, certain cancers, heart disease and stroke. Being underweight could also affect your health.

Most adults need to lose weight by eating fewer calories.

If you're trying to lose weight, aim to eat less and be more active. Eating a healthy, balanced diet can help you maintain a healthy weight.

Check whether you're a healthy weight by using the BMI healthy weight calculator.

Lose weight with the NHS weight loss plan, a 12-week weight loss guide that combines advice on healthier eating and physical activity.

If you're underweight, see underweight adults. If you're worried about your weight, ask your GP or a dietitian for advice.

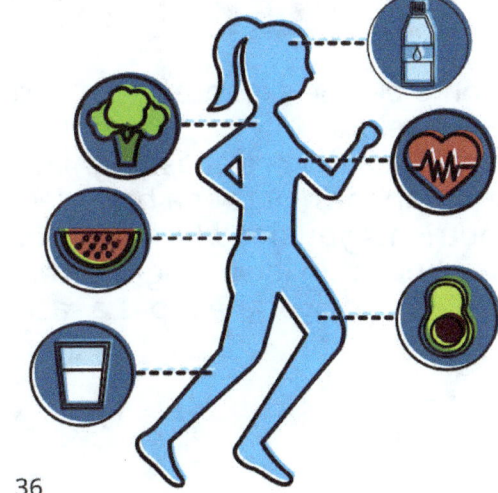

DO NOT GET THIRSTY

You need to drink plenty of fluids to stop you getting dehydrated. The government recommends drinking 6 to 8 glasses every day. This is in addition to the fluid you get from the food you eat.
All non-alcoholic drinks count, but water, lower fat milk and lower sugar drinks, including tea and coffee, are healthier choices.
Try to avoid sugary soft and fizzy drinks, as they're high in calories. They're also bad for your teeth.
Even unsweetened fruit juice and smoothies are high in free sugar.

Your combined total of drinks from fruit juice, vegetable juice and smoothies should not be more than 150ml a day, which is a small glass. Remember to drink more fluids during hot weather or while exercising.

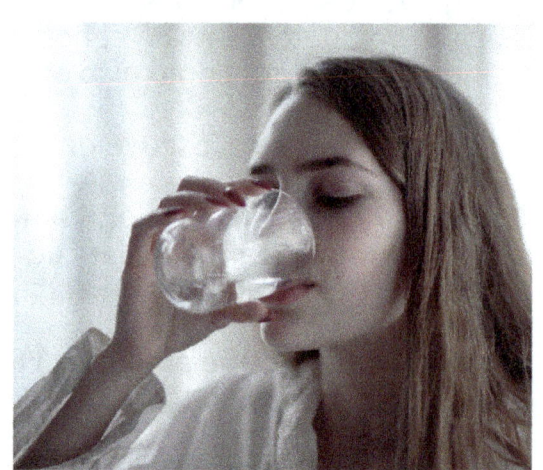

DO NOT SKIP BREAKFAST

Some people skip breakfast because they think it'll help them lose weight.
But a healthy breakfast high in fibre and low in fat, sugar and salt can form part of a balanced diet, and can help you get the nutrients you need for good health.
A wholegrain lower sugar cereal with semi-skimmed milk and fruit sliced over the top is a tasty and healthier breakfast.

NATURAL GUT HEALTH HACKS

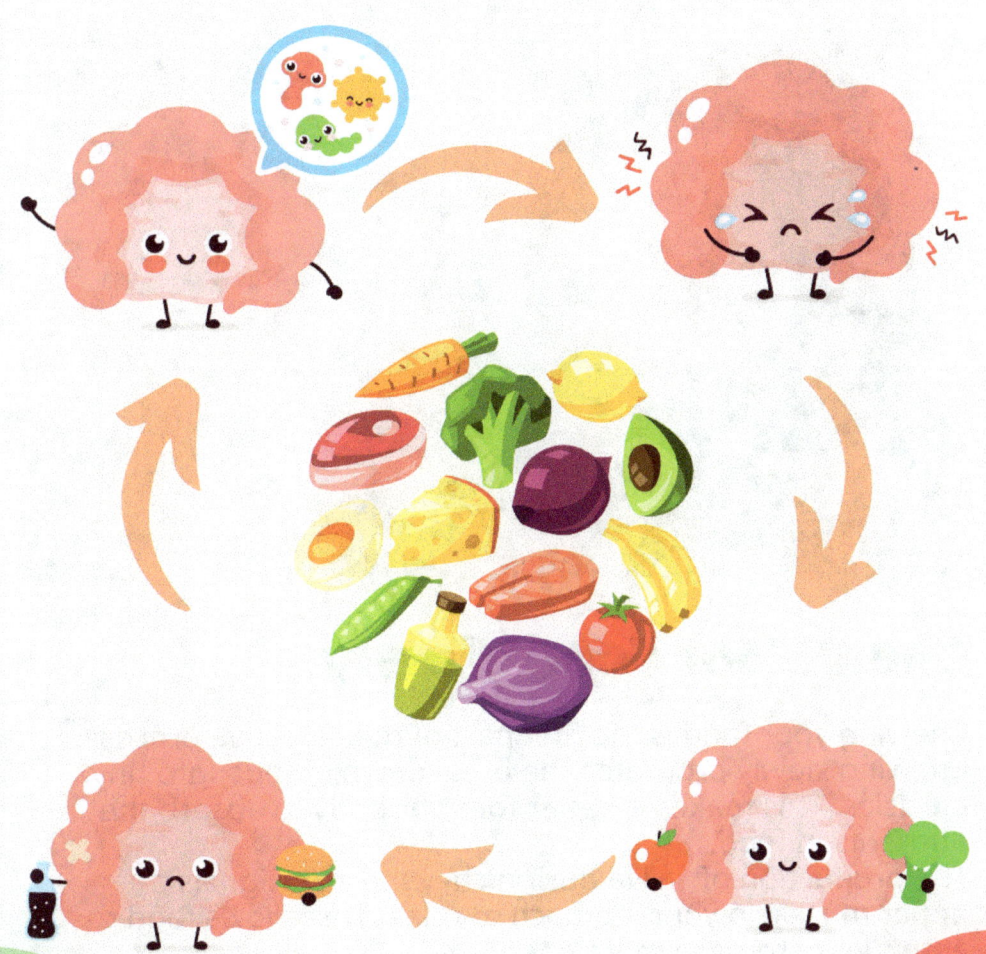

Drink Water in the Morning

Drinking water in the morning, especially before eating, can improve your digestion. Water helps break down the food you eat, which allows your body to absorb key nutrients. Drinking water also softens stools and can prevent constipation. What's more, drinking water before meals can help you feel fuller and avoid overeating.

Don't limit your water consumption to one part of the day, though! Sipping water throughout the day can keep you hydrated and support optimal digestion.

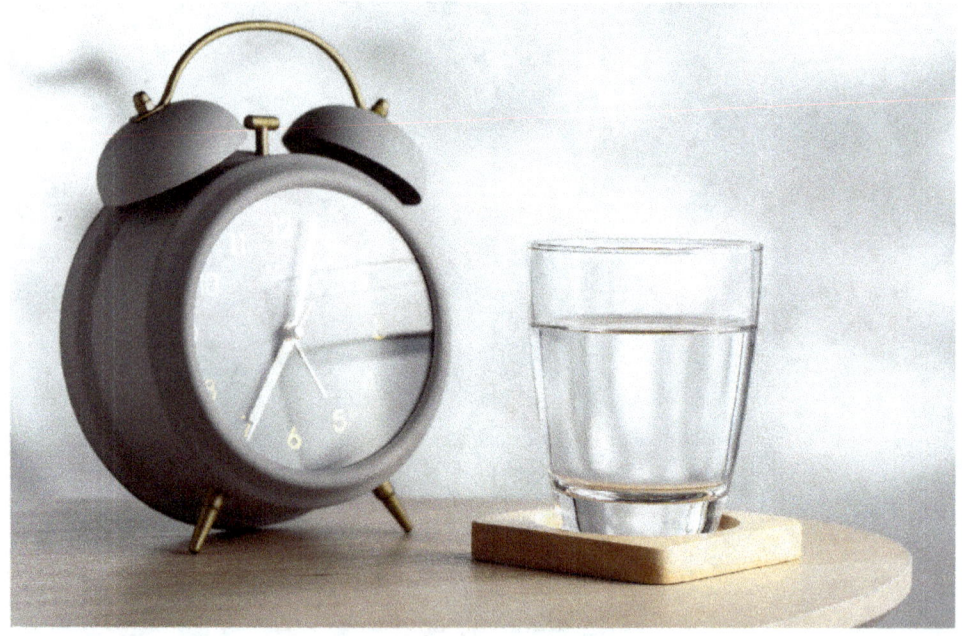

Chew Your Food Slowly

Chewing your food is the first part of the digestive process. Chewing slowly promotes the breakdown of food into tiny particles. This makes it easier for your body to absorb the nutrients in food.

The production of saliva during chewing also signals the upper muscle in your stomach to relax. This allows food to enter your stomach more easily.

Interestingly, one study found that chewing your food slowly can satisfy hunger cravings and reduce food consumption between meals.
But that's not all. Chewing your food slowly can also prevent you from swallowing excess air. This is a common cause of bloating.

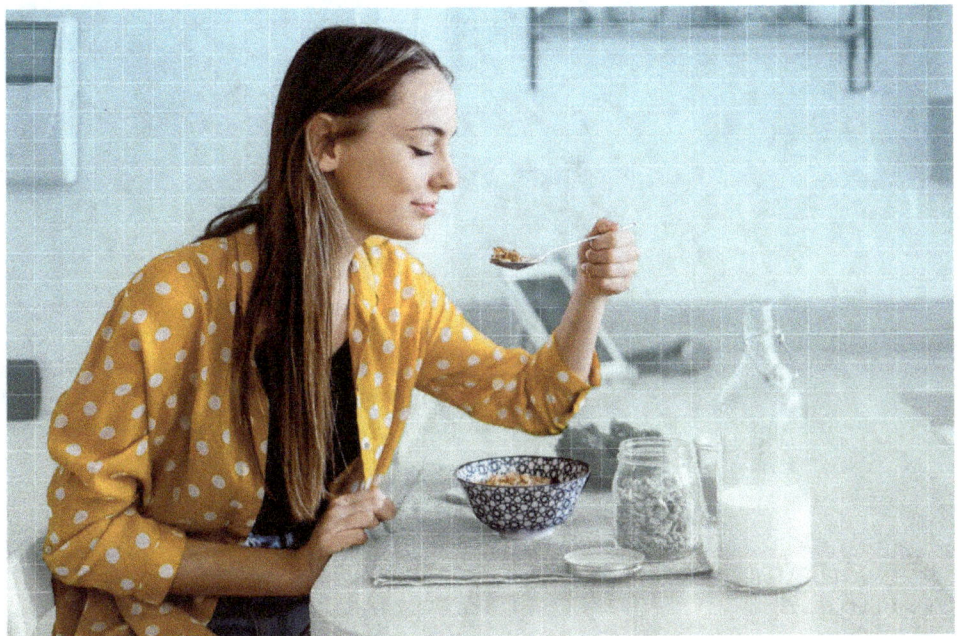

Drink Herbal Teas

Drinking herbal teas such as peppermint, chamomile, and ginger can treat many digestive symptoms and conditions.

Peppermint oil is a natural treatment for:
- Irritable bowel syndrome (IBS)
- Functional dyspepsia
- Childhood functional abdominal pain
- Post-operative nausea

Peppermint oil relaxes the smooth muscle in the gastrointestinal tract, reduces visceral pain, inhibits the growth of pathogens, and prevents gut inflammation. Chamomile can treat symptoms of inflammatory bowel disease (IBD). In fact, combining chamomile with myrrh and coffee charcoal can extend the remission phase in people with ulcerative colitis. Research shows this herbal blend is just as effective as the drug mesalazine.

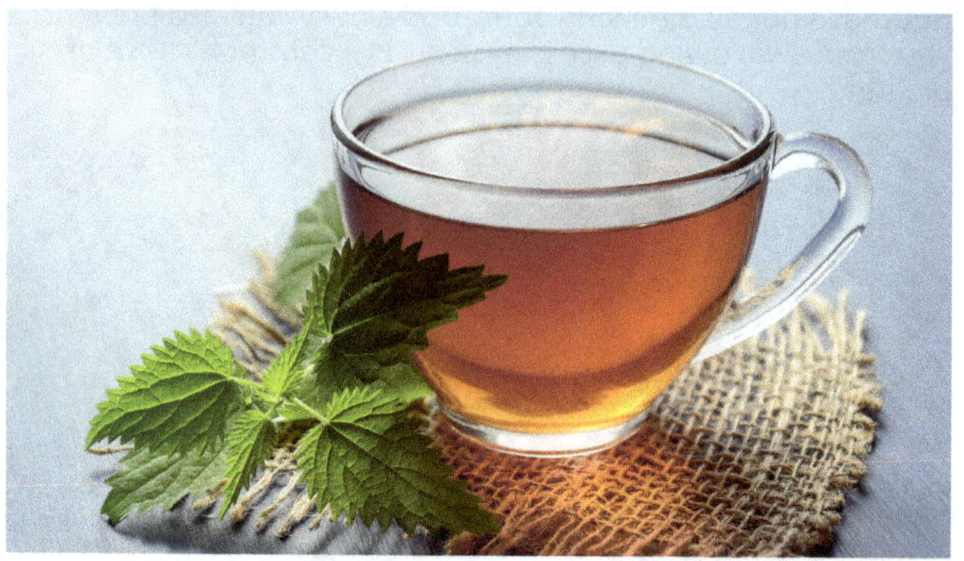

Ginger is a popular treatment for:
- Nausea
- Heartburn
- Flatulence
- Diarrhea
- Loss of appetite

Incredibly, ginger has anti-inflammatory, antioxidant, and anticancer properties that may also reduce the risk of gastrointestinal cancers. Studies show that ginger prevents the growth and spread of cancer cells in liver cancer, pancreatic cancer, colorectal cancer, and gastric cancer.

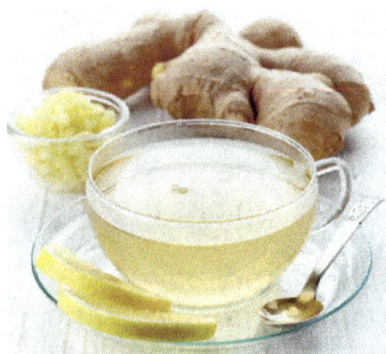
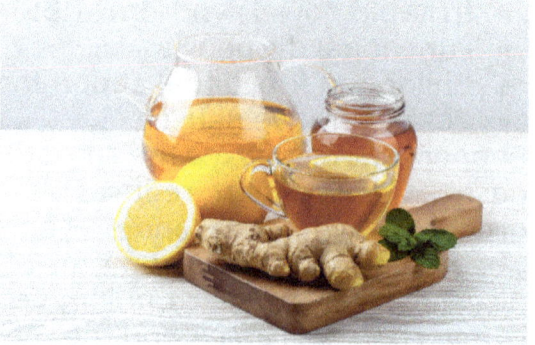

Consume Fruit by Itself

Consuming fruit by itself at least an hour before or after a meal can aid digestion and provide your body with a quick source of energy and nutrients. This is because fruit is the fastest digesting food.

Eating fruit with slow-digesting foods such as starches and proteins can slow down the digestive process. This can lead to uncomfortable symptoms such as bloating, indigestion, and flatulence.

However, you can still enjoy fruit with other foods on occasion. Green leafy vegetables also digest more quickly and can be eaten with fruit without any side effects. Being mindful of your food combination choices may help alleviate digestive problems.

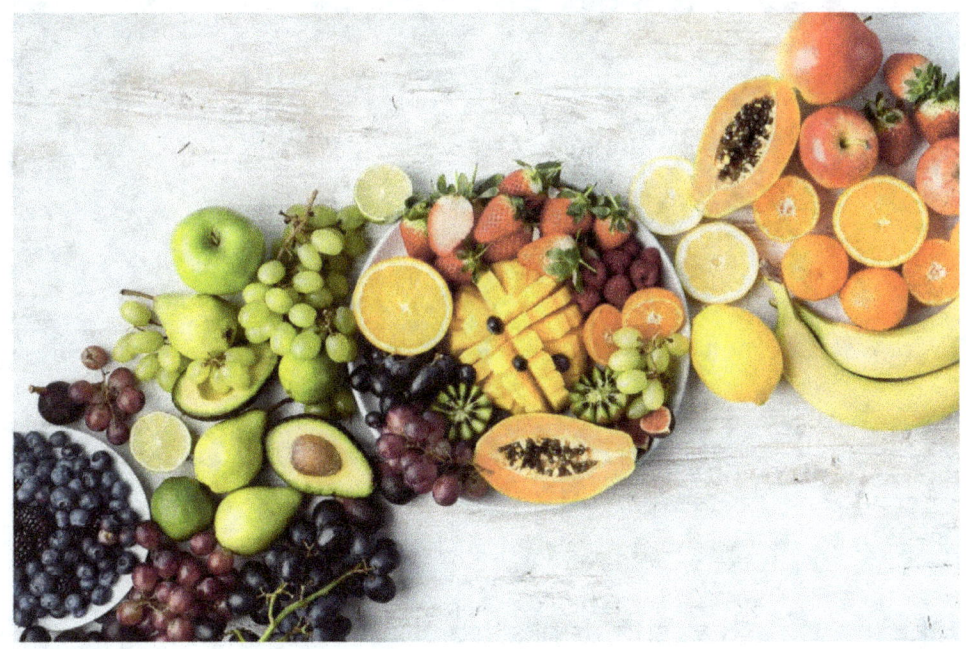

Eat Fiber-Rich Foods

Eating fiber-rich foods can naturally boost your gut health. Fiber is the indigestible plant material found in fruit, vegetables, legumes, grains, nuts, and seeds.

Fiber bulks up stools and makes them easier to pass. This can normalize bowel movements and prevent both constipation and diarrhea. Adding more fiber-rich foods to your diet can also reduce your risk of the following:
- Diverticulitis
- Hemorrhoids
- Gallstones
- Kidney stones
- Colon cancer
- Acid reflux
- Ulcers

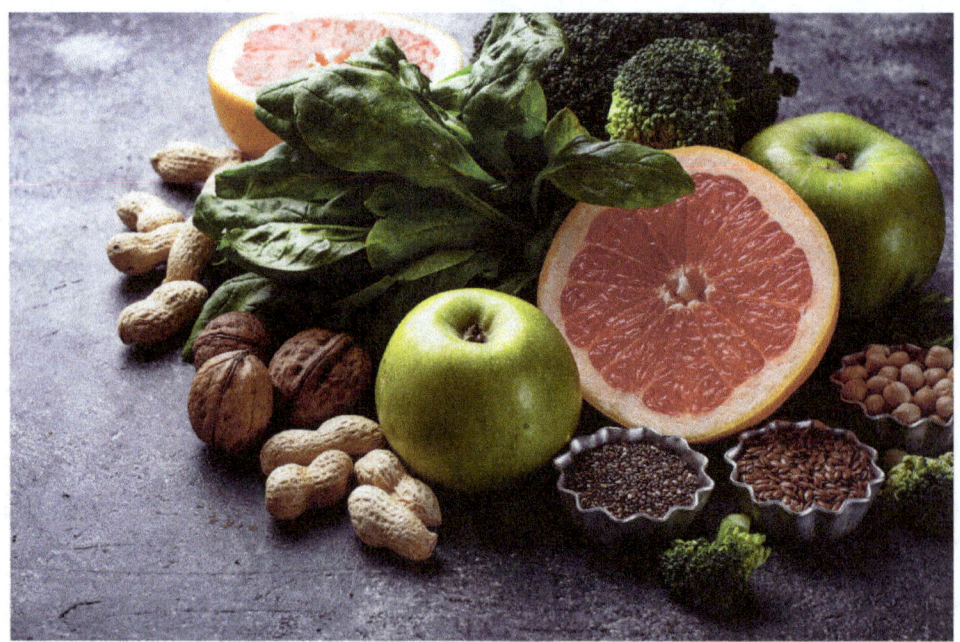

Ditch Junk Food

Junk foods such as soft drinks are often filled with high fructose corn syrup (HFCS), an artificial sugar made from corn syrup. HFCS contains unnaturally high levels of fructose that cause a stress response within the body and reduce insulin signaling in the liver.
Eating foods with HFCS can increase your risk of fatty liver disease, type 2 diabetes, and obesity.

Junk foods such as soft drinks are often filled with high fructose corn syrup (HFCS), an artificial sugar made from corn syrup. HFCS contains unnaturally high levels of fructose that cause a stress response within the body and reduce insulin signaling in the liver.
Eating foods with HFCS can increase your risk of fatty liver disease, type 2 diabetes, and obesity.

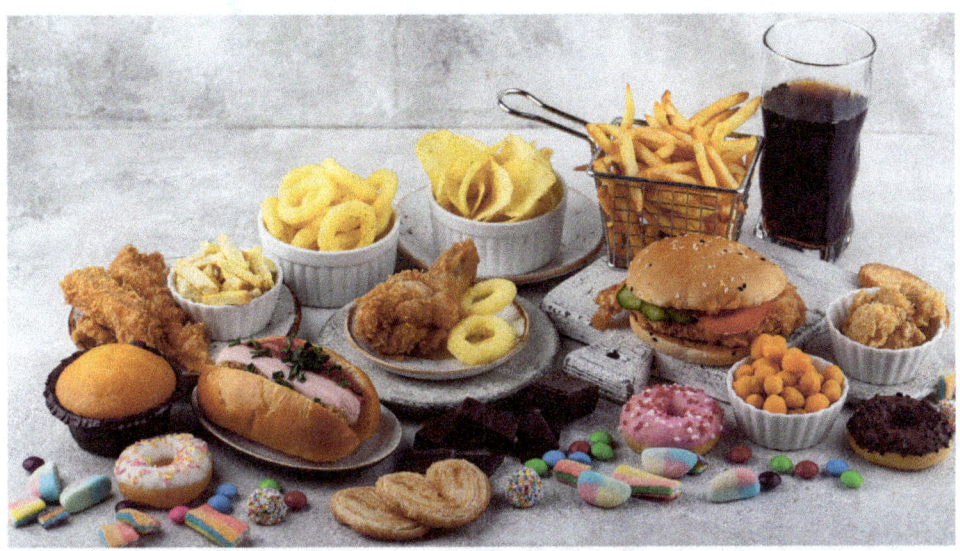

Additionally, junk foods usually lack fiber and other important nutrients. Eating too much junk food can lead to hard stools that are difficult to pass. Opting for whole, plant-based foods over junk foods can improve your digestion.

Stay Physically Active

Staying physically active has protective effects against chronic inflammatory diseases. Recent research shows that aerobic exercise can increase the diversity of healthy bacteria in the gut, which can benefit both gut and brain health.

Remarkably, aerobic exercise can reduce symptoms of IBS while also lowering levels of anxiety and depression.

Regular physical activity can also increase intestinal motility and regulate bowel movements.

PROBIOTICS SUPPORT THE INTESTINES

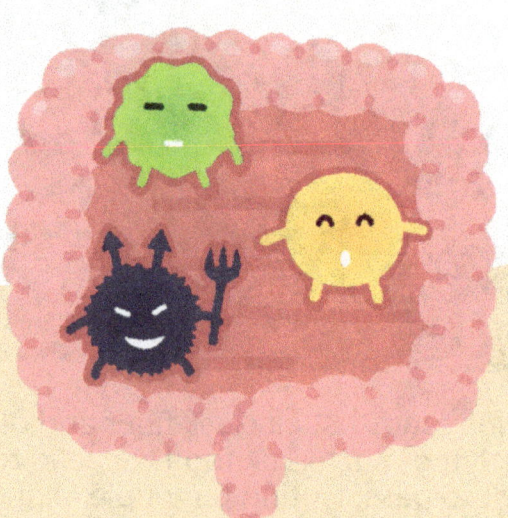

SUPPLEMENT PROBIOTICS

GUIDE TO CHOOSING THE BEST PROBIOTIC SUPPLEMENTS

Probiotics are getting a lot of attention lately. These live probiotic products have been documented to provide all sorts of health benefits related to gut function and more. However, not all foods high in probiotics are right for you.

If you're looking to use them to promote health, it's important to make sure you take the right probiotic supplements to get the results you're looking for.

What are probiotics?

Your gut contains bacteria acquired at birth and in later life through a process called colonization.
Many of these bacteria are considered beneficial. They have many functions including converting fiber into short-chain fatty acids, synthesizing certain vitamins, and supporting your immune system.
Using probiotics can help increase the number of these beneficial bacteria. The official definition of probiotics is, "a live microorganism that, when administered in appropriate amounts, confers a health benefit on the host".
Basically, probiotics are microorganisms that provide beneficial effects when used in appropriate amounts.
Probiotics can be taken in supplement form or from fermented foods like sauerkraut, kefir, and yogurt.
Probiotics should not be confused with prebiotics - a type of fiber that acts as a food source for the bacteria that live in your large intestine.
Certain probiotic products may have specific benefits. Probiotics that have been found to provide health benefits include different strains of Bifidobacterium, Lactobacillus and Saccharomyces. Many probiotic supplements contain

combinations of different strains in the same supplement. Research has shown that some strains of bacteria seem to be more effective than others in treating certain diseases. So you are more likely to get good results by taking a product that has been shown to achieve specific effects, such as controlling diarrhea.

Also, it is important that you consume the required amount of probiotics. Probiotics dosage is usually measured in colony-forming units (CFUs). In general, higher doses have been shown to produce the best results in most studies.

However, some products may be effective at dosages of 1–2 billion CFU per day, while others may require at least 20 billion CFU to achieve the desired effect.

Taking extremely high doses of probiotics has not been found to be harmful. One study showed that people taking doses up to 1.8 trillion CFUs per day experienced no problems.

However, it is expensive and does not seem to provide any additional benefits.

However, until now scientists did not know everything about probiotics. There is still much to be discovered about probiotics, although research has rapidly expanded over the past few years.

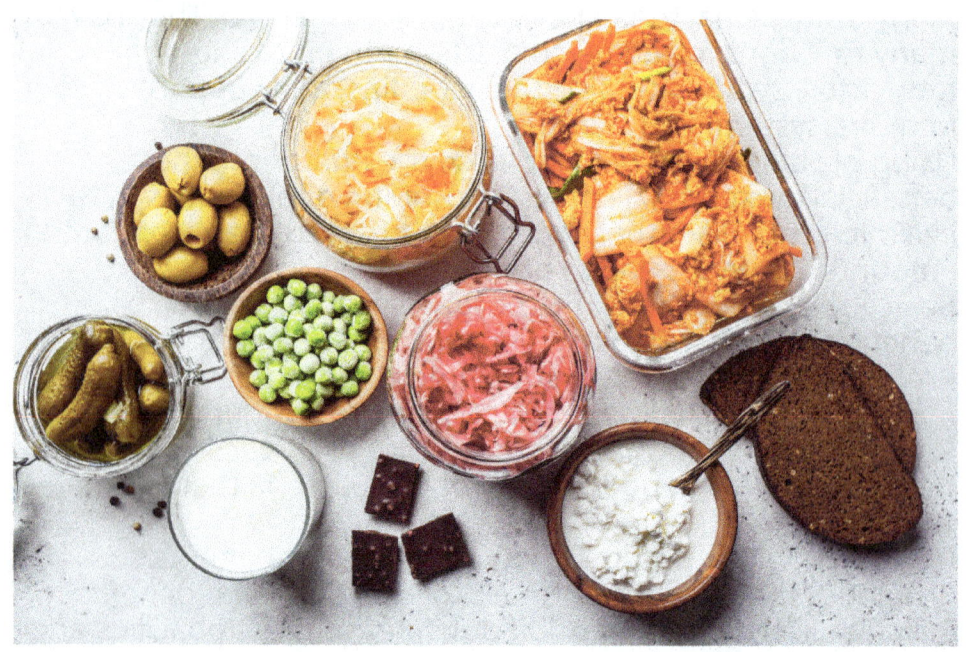

What are the effects of Probiotics supplements?

Probiotics can help relieve constipation Constipation is difficult, difficult, and infrequent bowel movements. Everyone experiences constipation at least once in their life, but for some it becomes a chronic problem.
Chronic constipation is most common in the elderly and bedridden adults, but it can also occur in children. Additionally, some people with irritable bowel syndrome also experience persistent constipation, which may be their main symptom.

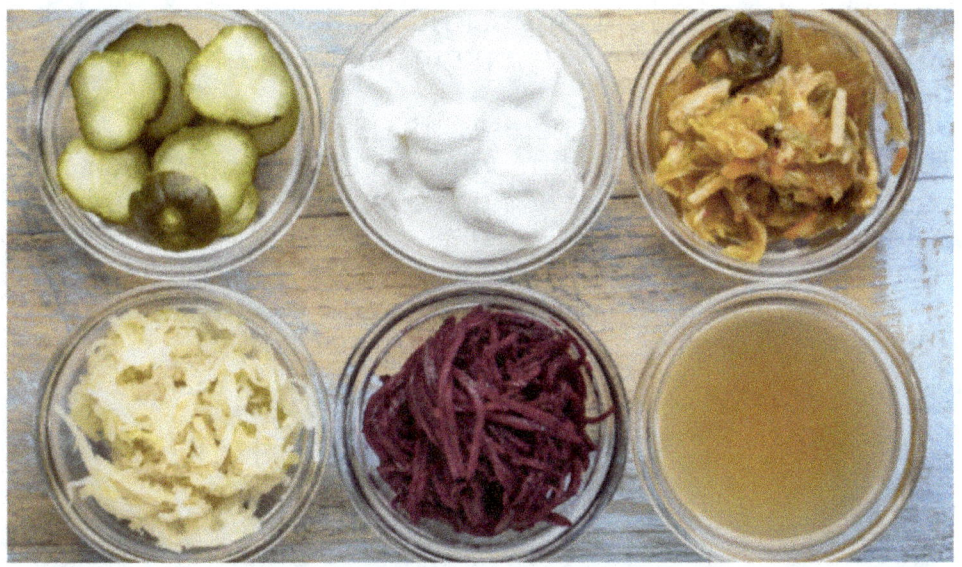

Common constipation treatments include laxatives and stool softeners. However, dietary changes and probiotic supplements have become an alternative in the treatment of constipation in recent years.
Several studies have shown that supplementing with certain strains of probiotics can relieve constipation in both adults and children. In a study comparing the effects of probiotics and prebiotics in children with irritable bowel syndrome, B. lactis significantly reduced constipation.
The probiotics group also had less belching, bloating and postprandial bloating than the prebiotics group.

Other probiotics that may improve constipation include B. longum, S. cerevisiae and a combination of L. acidophilus, L. plantarum, L. reuteri, L. rhamnosus and B. animalis.

Probiotics Can Improve IBS Symptoms Sometimes the main symptoms of IBS are not related to stool consistency or frequency. Instead, some patients frequently experience bloating, gas, and bloating. gas, nausea and lower abdominal pain.

A review based on 19 studies found that while some patients reported improvement in IBS symptoms when taking probiotics, the results varied between individuals. The researchers were unable to determine which probiotics were most effective.

Also, because the symptoms of irritable bowel syndrome are so varied, sometimes one symptom improves while others do not.

For example, a study of people with IBS primarily due to constipation found that although S. cerevisiae improved constipation, it did not have much of an effect on abdominal pain or discomfort.

In another study, participants with irritable bowel syndrome predominantly with diarrhea were given a product supplement containing strains of Lactobacillus,

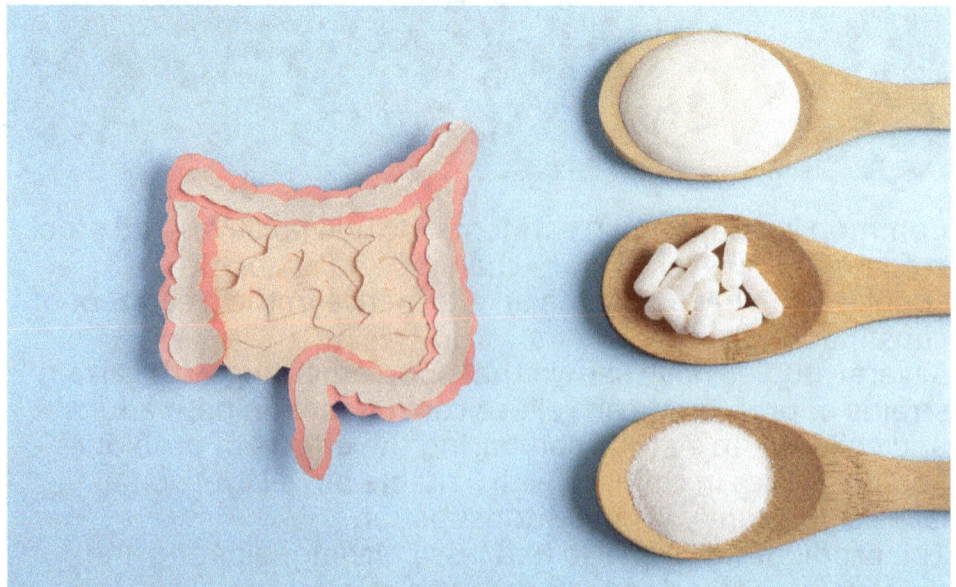

Bifidobacterium, and Streptococcus. Results showed that bowel movements and consistency did not improve, but symptoms of bloating did.
Another study showed a significant reduction in pain and bloating during treatment with the above probiotic product. Researchers believe that probiotics lead to an increase in melatonin, which is a hormone involved in digestive function.

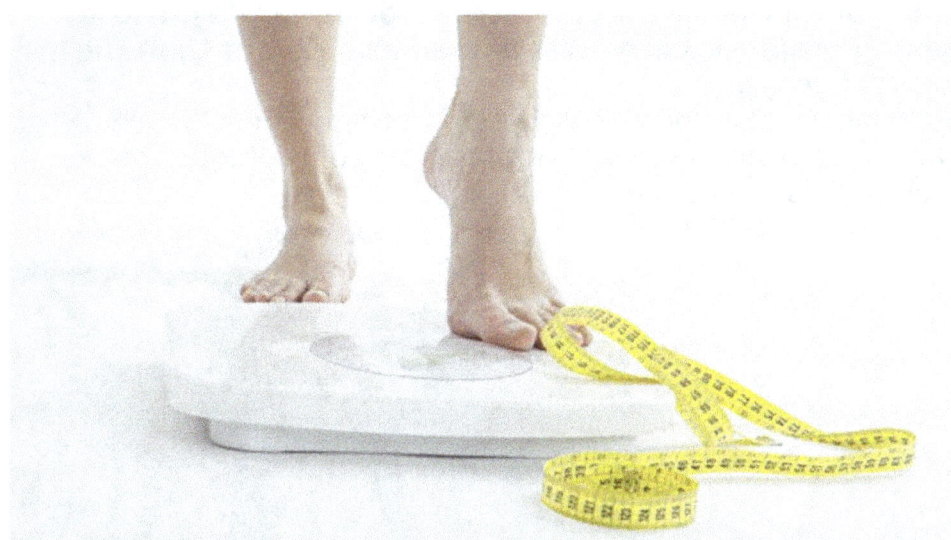

Probiotics can help you lose weight There is growing evidence that the balance of your gut bacteria can have a profound effect on your body weight. Several studies have shown that taking probiotic supplements can be helpful in losing weight and staying healthy.
Animal and human studies have found that certain strains of bacteria can reduce the amount of fat and calories absorbed by the gut, promote a healthy balance of gut bacteria, and reduce weight and belly fat.
According to a 2014 analysis based on several studies, probiotics that appear to be effective for fat loss include Lactobacillus rhamnosus, Lactobacillus gasseri and a combination of Lactobacillus rhamnosus and Bifidobacterium lactis.
In one study, obese men who were given L. gasseri for 12 weeks experienced a significant reduction in body weight and body fat, specifically up to 8.5% reduction in belly fat.

In another study, obese women who were given L. rhamnosus for three weeks lost twice as much weight as those given a placebo. Interestingly, they continued to lose weight during the study's maintenance period, while the placebo group gained weight.

Probiotic supplements can also help limit weight gain when you consume a lot of calories. In a 4-week study, thin young men ate 1,000 extra calories per day. Those taking probiotics products gained less weight than the control group.

However, researchers feel there is not enough evidence to draw firm conclusions about the effects of probiotics on weight loss at this time.

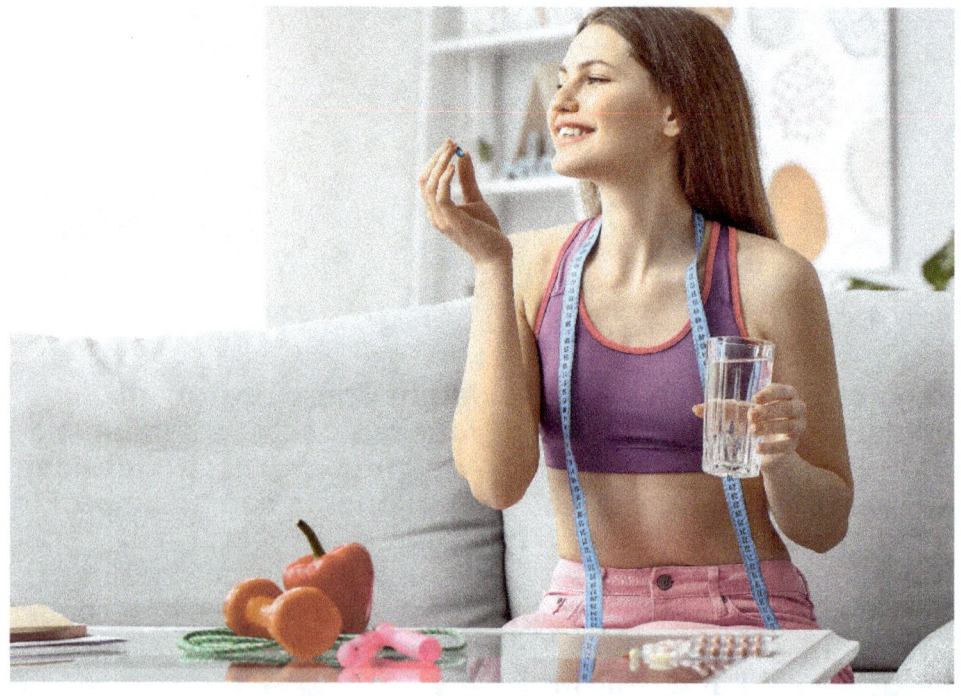

Probiotics to support brain health Gut and brain health are closely linked. Bacteria in the large intestine digest and ferment fiber into short-chain fatty acids that nourish the intestines. Research has shown that these compounds may also benefit the brain and nervous system.

A review of 38 animal and human studies found that various probiotics improved symptoms of depression, autism, anxiety, obsessive-compulsive disorder and poor memory.

The bacterial strains commonly used in these studies were Bifidobacterium longum, Bifidobacterium breve, Bifidobacterium infantis, Lactobacillus helveticus and Lactobacillus rhamnosus.

Probiotics appear to be effective for both generalized anxiety and anxiety related to specific causes. One study found that when nasopharyngeal cancer patients took probiotics for two weeks before surgery, they had lower blood stress hormone levels and a 48 percent reduction in anxiety.

In other studies, probiotics have been shown to improve overall mood and reduce sadness in healthy individuals and in patients with chronic fatigue syndrome.

Probiotic supplements can also help you cope with depression, even those with major depressive disorder. In an 8-week study of patients with major depression, those taking L. casei, L. acidophilus, and B. bifidum experienced significant reductions in depression.

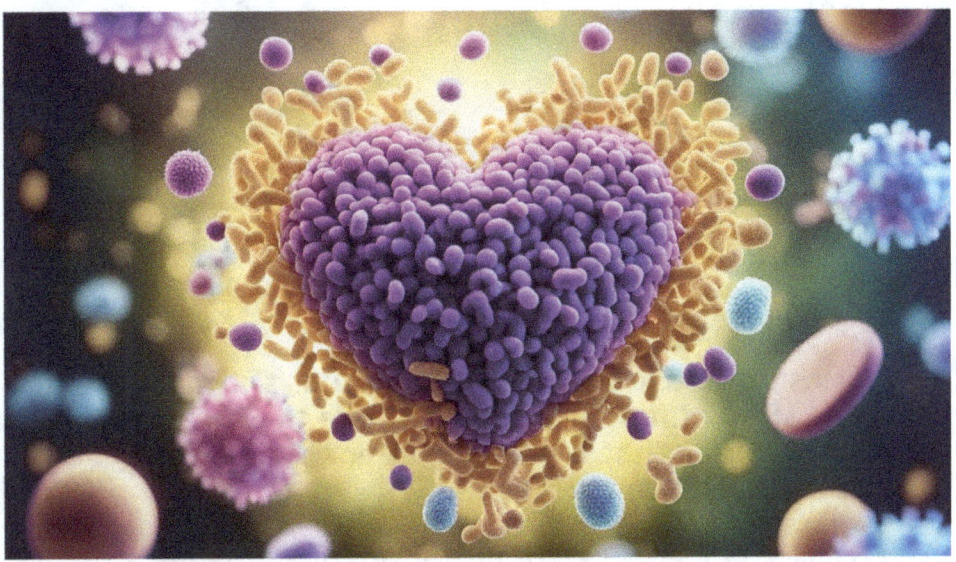

Probiotics May Improve Heart Health Taking probiotics may help reduce the risk of cardiovascular disease. Some studies have found that certain strains of bacteria in yogurt or probiotic supplements can lead to beneficial changes in markers of heart health. Those beneficial changes include lowering "bad" LDL cholesterol and increasing "good" HDL cholesterol.

Specific strains of bacteria that are thought to be effective in lowering cholesterol levels include Lactobacillus acidophilus, Lactobacillus reuteri, and Bifidobacterium longum.

An analysis of 14 studies found probiotics to moderate LDL cholesterol, slightly increase HDL, and lower triglycerides. There may be several processes responsible for these effects, including changes in fat metabolism and decreased absorption of cholesterol in the gut.

A review based on 9 controlled studies found a slight decrease in blood pressure in people taking probiotics. However, more than eight weeks of use with a higher dose of 10 billion CFU per day has been found to have a significant effect.

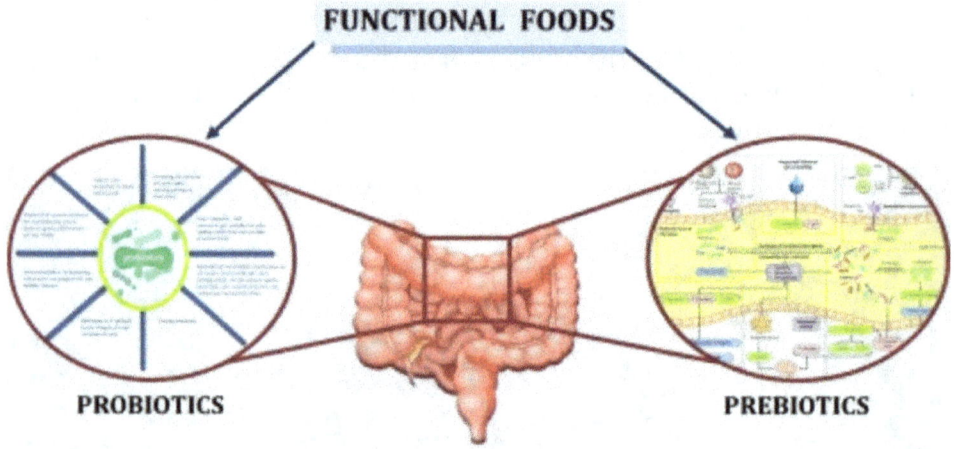

Probiotics for Boosting Immunity Studies show that taking probiotic supplements can help change the balance of gut bacteria in a way that enhances defenses against infections, allergies, and cancer.

Especially strains of Lactobacillus GG, Lactobacillus gasseri, Lactobacillus crispatus, Bifidobacterium bifidum and Bifidobacterium longum. These strains of bacteria seem to reduce the risk of respiratory disease and eczema in children, as well as reduce the risk of urinary tract infections in adult women. In addition, probiotics have been shown to reduce inflammation, which is a risk factor for many different diseases.

In one study, older adults consumed a mixture of Lactobacillus gasseri, Bifidobacterium bifidum and

Bifidobacterium longum or a placebo for three weeks. After probiotic supplementation, inflammatory markers decreased, anti-inflammatory markers increased, and the gut microbial balance became similar to that of the gut microbiota in young, healthy individuals.

Some probiotic products can also help prevent gingivitis or gum infections. One 14-day study looked at adults who didn't brush and floss while given either a Lactobacillus brevis supplement or a placebo. The results showed that gingivitis progressed faster in the placebo group, suggesting that probiotics helped protect against infection.

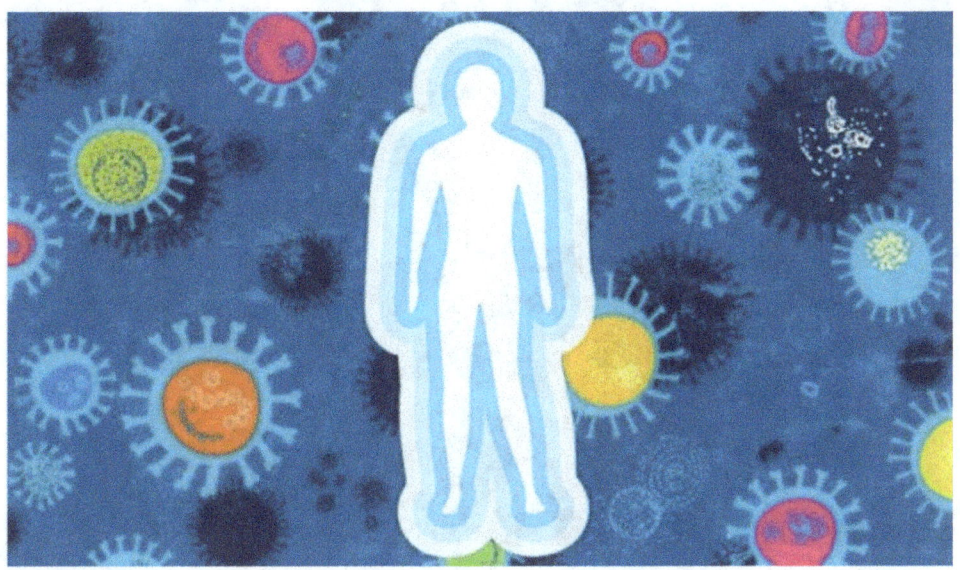

Probiotics for General Health In addition to using probiotics for specific diseases and conditions, you can also take probiotics to promote overall health.

A recent study performed in healthy adults found that taking Bifidobacterium bifidum for four weeks increased production of beneficial short-chain fatty acids. There's also some evidence that probiotics can reduce inflammation that often occurs as you age.

Of course, along with taking probiotics supplements you also have to make sure you're eating a healthy diet and practicing other health-promoting behaviors. Without taking measures as a whole, you can't expect probiotics to give you much benefit.

Also, while probiotics are safe for most people, they can be harmful to people who are very sick or have compromised immune systems, including those with HIV or AIDS. .
Having a healthy gut microbiome is extremely important. Although research is still ongoing, probiotics appear to have beneficial effects on a number of different health conditions and may also support better overall health. Taking the right probiotics product right can help you target specific health problems and improve your overall health and quality of life.

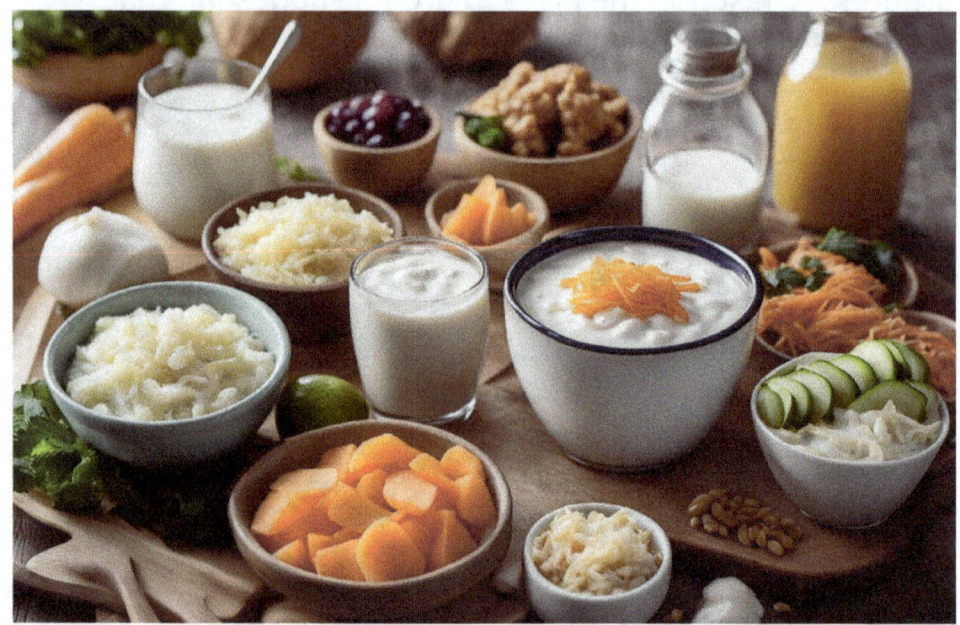

PROBIOTIC DISRUPTORS

Your Out-of-Whack Schedule

Turns out, your microbiome is impacted by that midnight snack.
Late-night eating can throw off our natural circadian rhythm and promotes an imbalance in the microbiome, according to some recent research.
So if you're staying up late, spending more time inside sitting in front of the TV and indulging in not-so-healthy comfort foods a little too often, your gut could be feeling it.

Empty Supermarket Shelves and Processed Foods

In times when supermarket shelves are sometimes empty and restocking is unpredictable, you may find yourself reaching for things your gut isn't used to digesting.
Instead of the normal selection of gut-friendly fresh fruits and vegetables, you may be relying on more processed and packaged foods that oftentimes contain excess sugar, fat and salt, along with refined grains and genetically engineered ingredients.
An added wellness tidbit of information? Many nonorganic corn and soy ingredients found in thousands of ultra-processed foods are grown from genetically modified seeds, and those could be foods you're typically not used to eating or your gut's not accustomed to.
Interestingly, Danish scientists found what they termed "excessive" levels of glyphosate in U.S. soy, and independent testing routinely IDs glyphosate in U.S. processed foods.

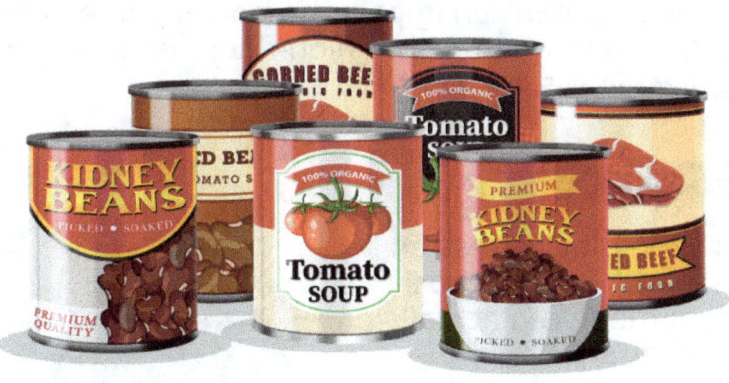

Excessive Sugar Intake

Eating too much added sugars, including man-made sweeteners like high-fructose corn syrup, can impact the gut in ways that can throw you out of balance.
Opt for small amounts of stevia or raw honey or real maple syrup when you need an occasional sweetener, but be careful not to overdo it.

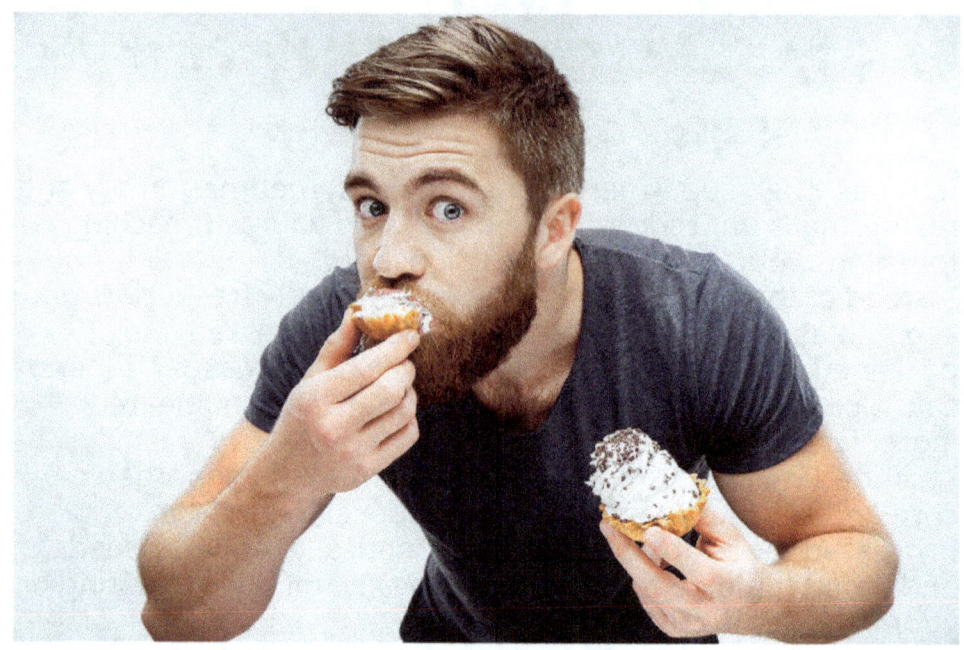

Overloading on Grains and Gluten

Eating too much gluten can impact the gut for some people, while opting for a low-gluten, but high-fiber diet seems to promote gut wellness, in general.

Excess Stress

We all know too much stress on a daily basis is bad. But too much fight-or-flight mode can actually agitate the body's gut microbiome. Along with probiotics, it can be a wise move to pick up some other stress support supplements.

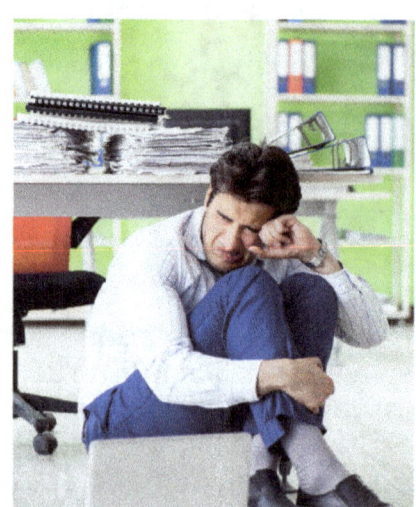

GUT-SUPPORT HACKS

Source as Many Gut-Friendly Foods as You Can

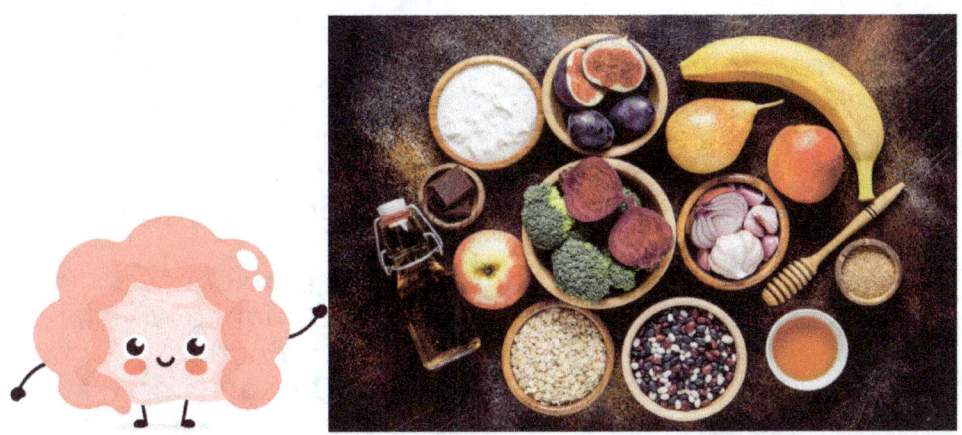

Look for digestive tract-friendly foods and drinks, including probiotic foods like sauerkraut, kombucha and kefir.
Other gut-friendly foods and drinks include green tea, coconut water, sprouted seeds, avocados, olive oil, coconut oil, bone broth, ghee, cooked vegetables, fiber-rich fruits and made-from-scratch soups and stews.
Here's an easy recipe to get started making your own fermented foods at home on the cheap.
To make your own sauerkraut, follow these simple steps:
- Clean one head of cabbage and chop it into small pieces or shreds.
- Add 1½ to 2 teaspoons of sea salt.
- Massage the two together for several minutes in a large bowl so some of the water is released from the cabbage. (Keep it, you'll need it!)
- Pack mixture into a quart-sized glass jar with a tight-fitting lid.
- After waiting for several days or weeks, depending on conditions, you've got homemade sauerkraut containing live probiotics, fiber and other nutrients.

Use 'Tough' Probiotics for Tough Times

In addition to a gut-friendly diet and lifestyle, many people choose to take gut support to the next level using probiotic supplements.

Here's the thing: The point of probiotic supplements is to make it to your intestines to offer gut and digestive health support. But many strains of probiotic products require refrigeration and experience "die off" by body temperature and acids before even making it to the GI tract.

This is why soil-based organisms (SBOs), or supplements like SBO Probiotics, come into play.

Unlike more fragile refrigeration-required probiotics, "survivable" soil-based probiotics are built tough to withstand the heat, acid and harsh journey from your mouth to your intestines. All of this happens even when they are stored at room temperature.

SBO Probiotics, for instance, contains many of the same soil-derived strains your great-grandparents and ancestors ingested when they enjoyed fruits and veggies straight out of the garden. This SBO Probiotic version contains those same strains, but is formulated to maximize quality.

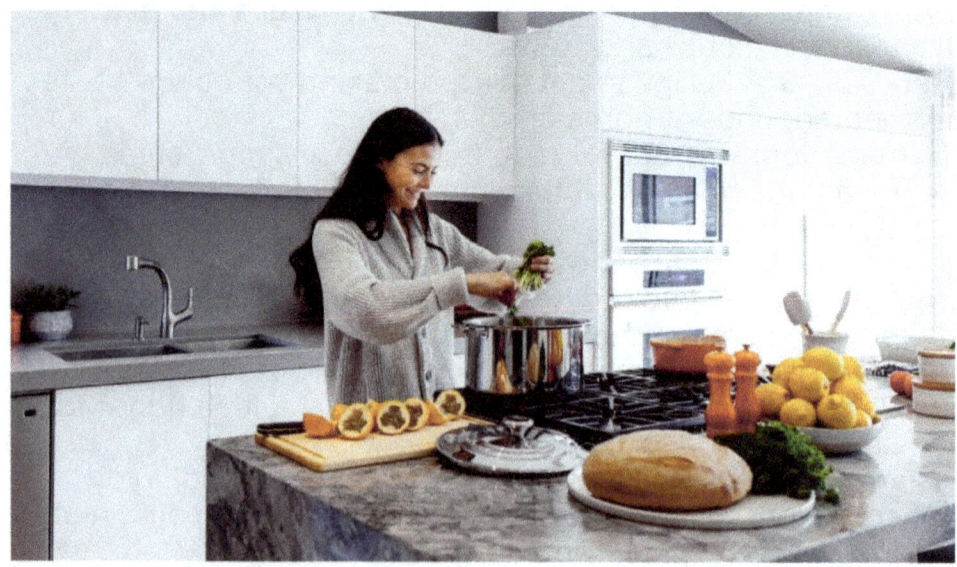

Clean Up Your Diet

Here's a list of foods to limit or completely avoid:
- Processed foods: fried foods, baked goods, fast food, convenience meals
- Refined carbs: white bread, pasta, crackers, chips, tortillas
- Processed meats: bacon, salami, bologna, beef jerky, lunch meats
- Sugary drinks: soda, fruit juice, sweet tea, sports drinks, energy drinks
- Added sugar: high-fructose corn syrup, table sugar, agave nectar, molasses

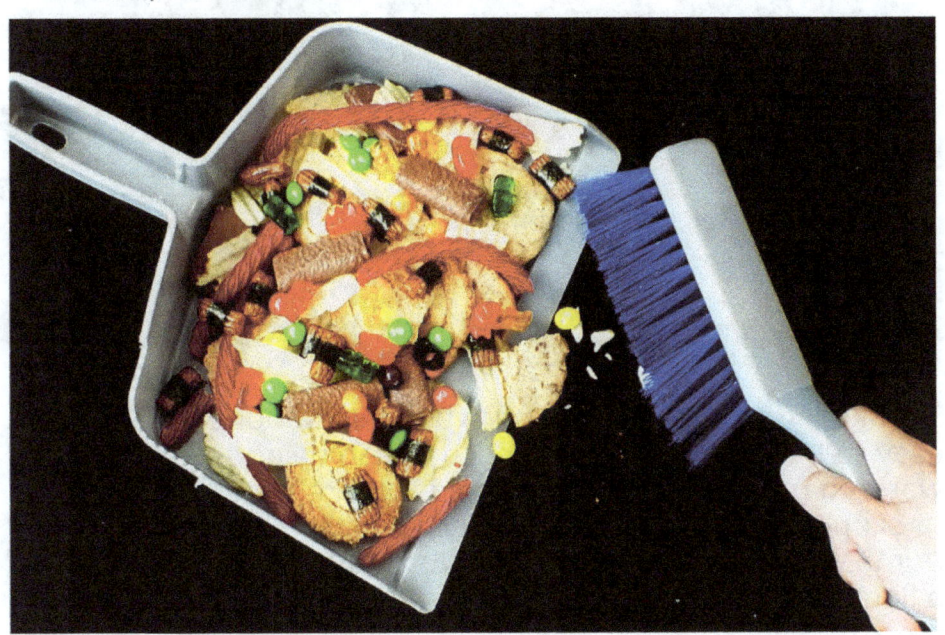

Start Supporting Your Gut with Supportive Ingredients

Between stress, diet choices and an inactive lifestyle, our guts can take a beating. But one time-treasured ingredient people have turned to for centuries is bone broth. There's a reason moms around the world still give their kids chicken soup when they're needing a boost.

Traditionally used for centuries, chicken bone broth inherently features glucosamine, chondroitin, hyaluronic acid and 19 amino acids to bring whole food-based gut support.

The only downside is it does take about a day or more to make bone broth, and that batch doesn't always last very long.

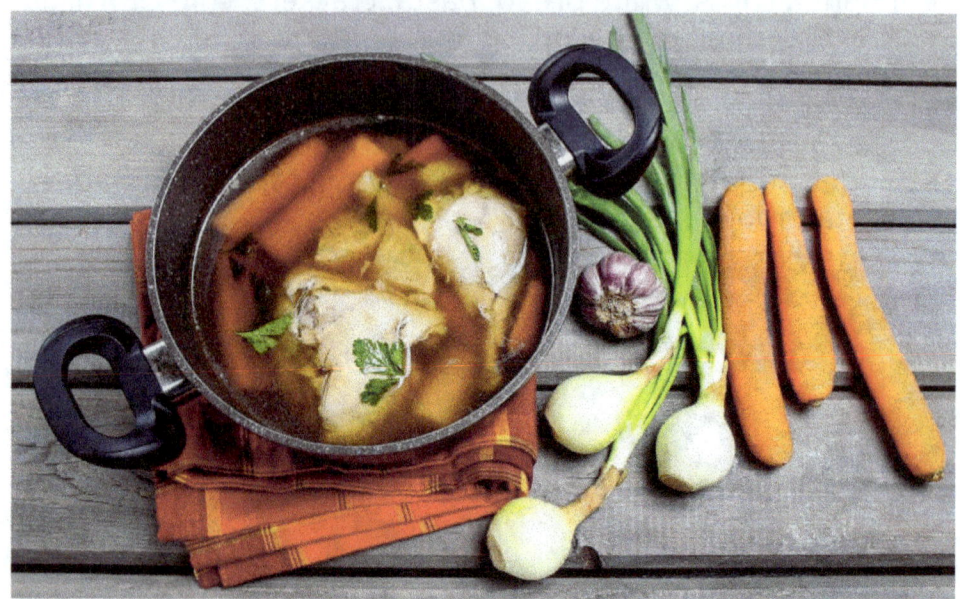

Thankfully, you can now get the benefits of bone broth in an easy-to-use instant powder mix that can be added to hot water to make a savory homemade chicken broth in seconds, or slipped into rice, soups, sauces and stews for a wellness bump with each scoop. Ancient Nutrition also recently created a line of sipping bone broths.

'Weight Train' Your Diaphragm to Get Your Body Out of Stress Mode

The first step to dialing down your body's overreaction to stress is to retrain the body to breathe the way it's meant to: diaphragmatically.

For most folks, everyday stress leads to habitual shallow "chest breathing," where secondary respiratory muscles like the scalenes, pectoralis minor and sternocleidomastoid muscles take over the diagram muscle's main job.

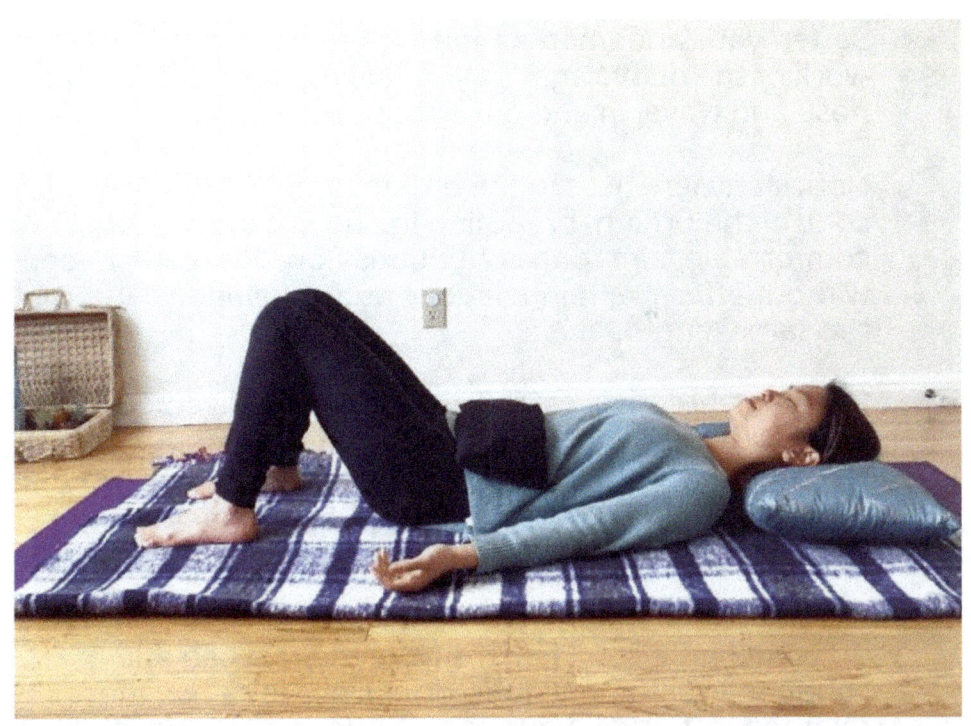

This promotes a vicious cycle, keeping the body tethered to fight-flight-or-freeze mode while deterring it entering "rest and digest" mode.

A simple way to work with improving diaphragmatic breathing is "sandbag breathing" using a five-pound bag of rice:

1. Lying on your back with a thin cushion under your head, extend the legs long, resting on the floor, placing your arms on the floor along your sides with the palms facing up. For lower-back support, place a rolled up blanket behind the backs of the knees.

2. Close your eyes and start envisioning the diaphragm muscle underneath your lungs and heart. As you inhale, picture the muscle turning into a dome, or parachute, drawing down toward the navel as your lungs fill with air and your belly rises.

3. On an exhale, visualize the diaphragm rising back up.

4. Soften your abdomen as you continue to visualize the work of the diaphragm as you feel the breath enter the nose and travel in and out of the body.

5. Notice any jerkiness in the breath, and without trying to control the breath, breathing in and out of the nose if comfortable, aim for a continuous flow of breath, deep without effort, with inhalations and exhalations about the same length.

6. Once this breath is established, place the five-pound bag of rice across the abdomen to start strength training your diaphragm muscle. As you inhale, the diagram draws down, belly lifts, ribs expand, then let it go on the exhale.

7. As long as the weighted breathing is comfortable, start off with 5 minutes. Then, remove the rice bag and continue breathing diaphragmatically for a few more minutes resting on your back. Notice any changes you may or may not experience.

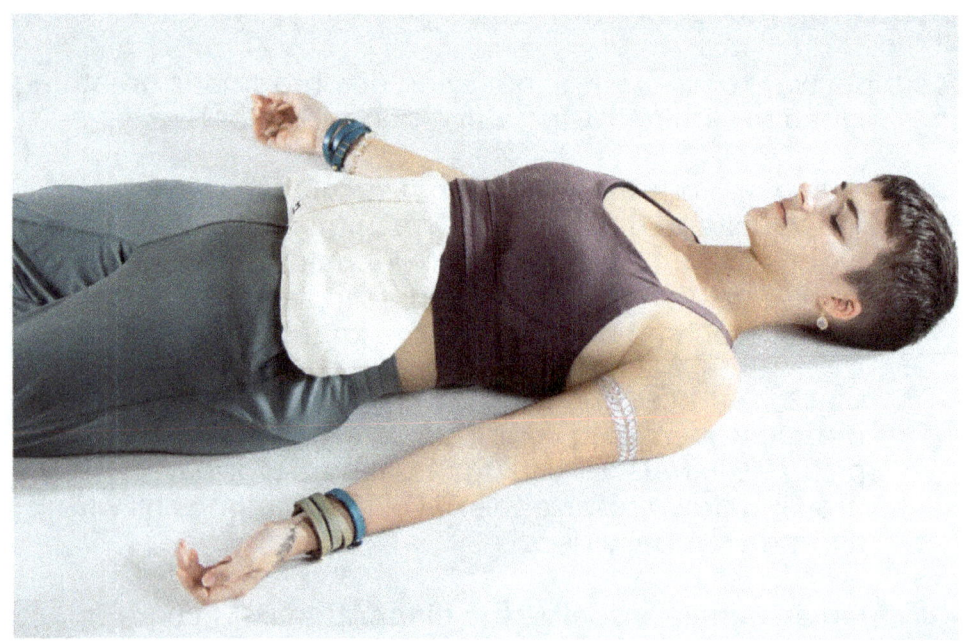

SURPRISING LIFESTYLE HABITS

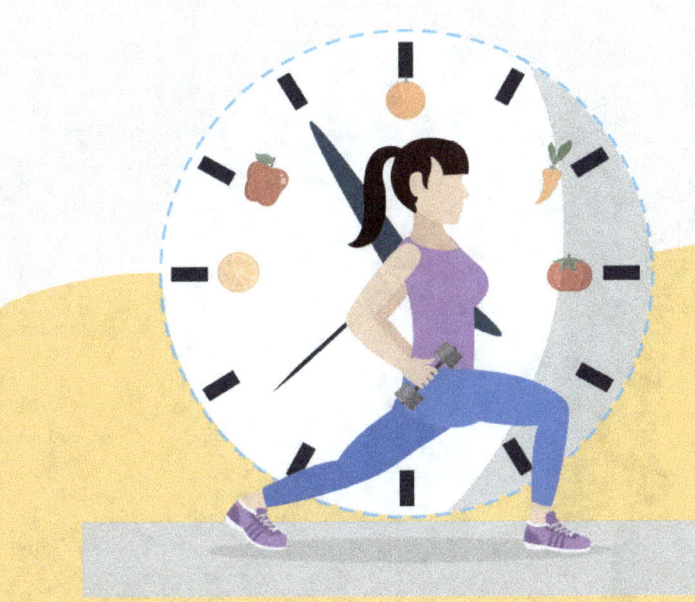

It's true that active cultures are good for you. However, improving your gut health goes beyond snacking on Greek yogurt. Exercise, sleep, mindfulness, meditation, and other lifestyle habits have just as much impact on your health as dietary choices.

As research unfolds about the gut-brain axis, we see further evidence of the relationship between mental health and the health of the gut microbiome. The gut microbiome reflects the community of little critters living in the gastrointestinal tract (a.k.a. the gut).

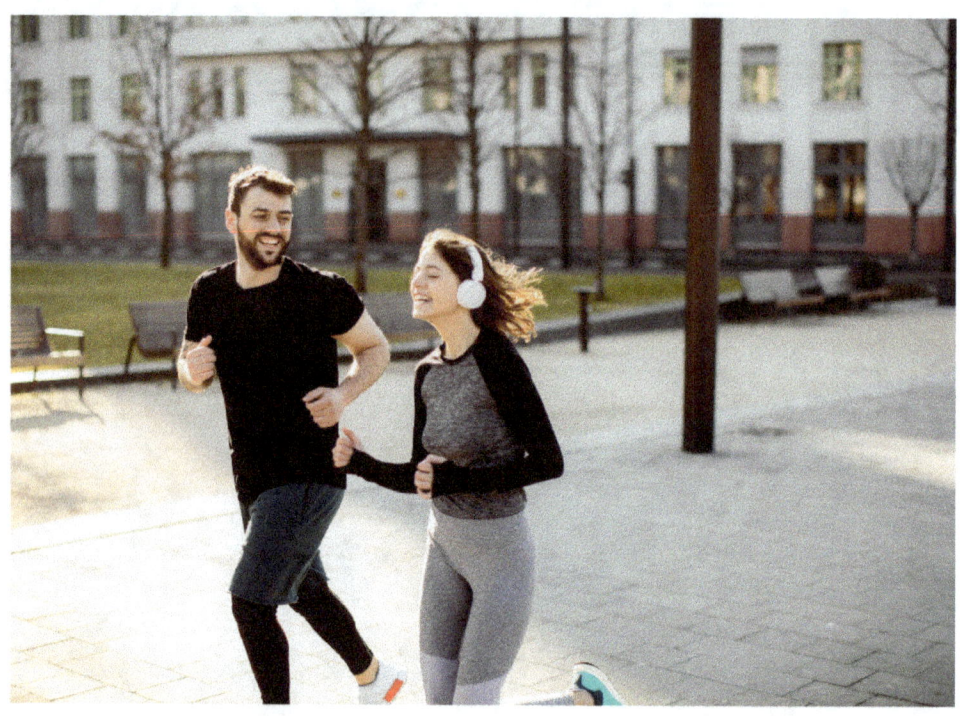

This community is important in maintaining an environment in the gut that supports the production of neurotransmitters, serotonin, epinephrine, dopamine, and norepinephrine. Neurotransmitters are essential for regulating mood, behavior, and stress response.

On the other hand, our mental health and habits affect the function of the gut. For example, when we are sleep deprived or live in a stressful environment, the gut microbiome can suffer. Below are 10 examples of how healthy lifestyle habits affect the population and balance of the gut microbiome.

MEDITATE 10 MINUTES EACH DAY TO RELAX THE MIND AND BODY. STRESS IS HARMFUL TO THE GUT MICROBIOME AND MINDFULNESS AND MEDITATION CAN HELP TO REDUCE STRESS AND SUPPORT GUT HEALTH.

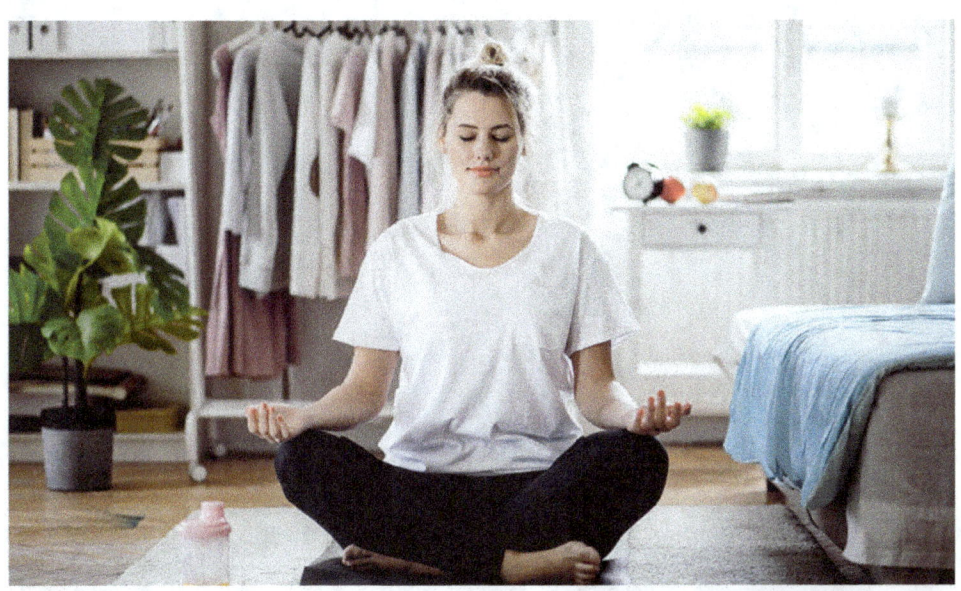

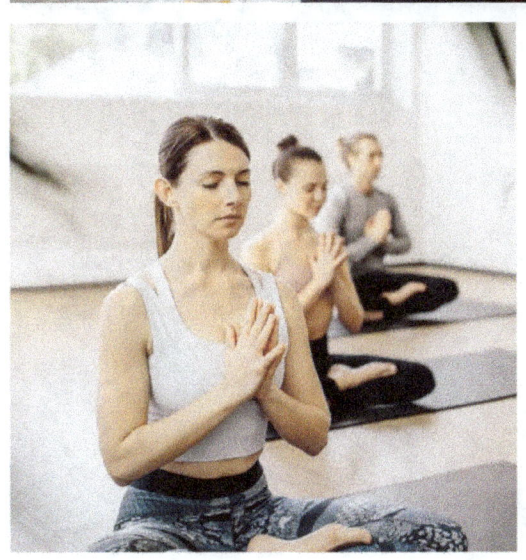

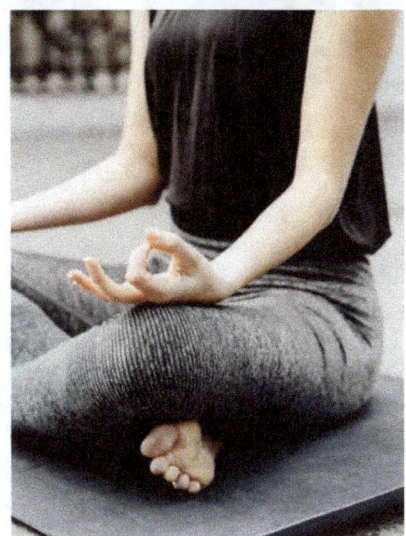

SLEEP IN A ROOM THAT IS 64°-69° F (17.8°-20.6° C) TO SUPPORT SLEEP QUALITY. SLEEP LOSS CAN NEGATIVELY AFFECT THE RATIOS OF GUT BACTERIA AND CAUSE OTHER HEALTH PROBLEMS.

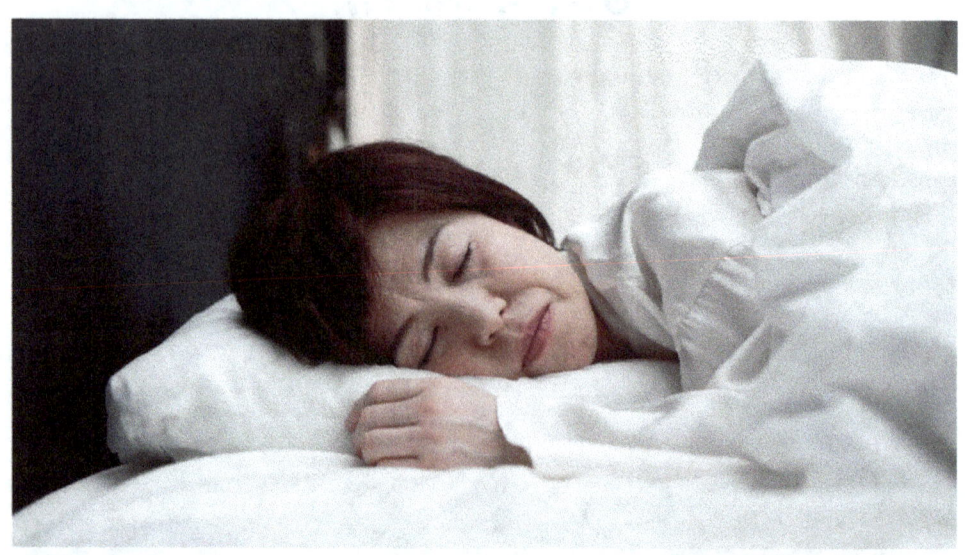

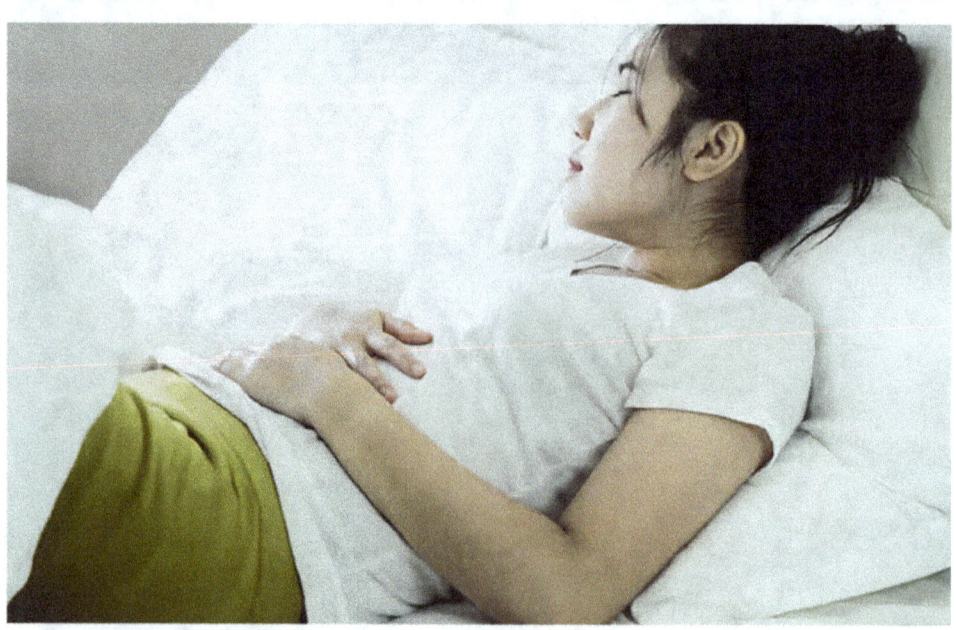

AVOID USING ANTI-INFLAMMATORY DRUGS AND/OR OPIOIDS (WHEN POSSIBLE). OVERUSE OF ANTI-INFLAMMATORY DRUGS AND/OR OPIOIDS CAN HAVE A NEGATIVE EFFECT ON THE HEALTH OF THE GUT MICROBIOME.

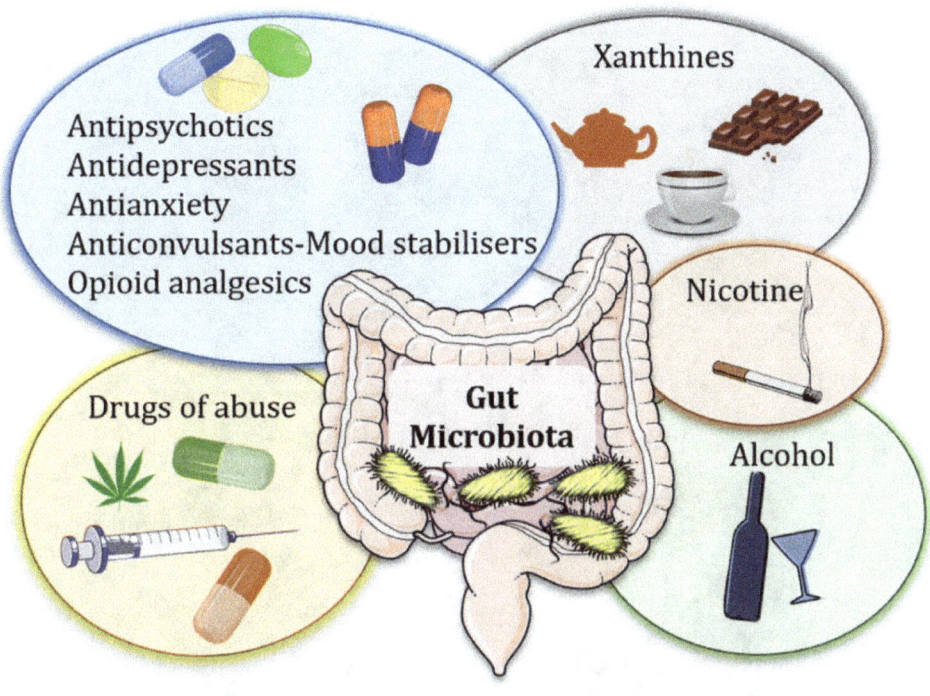

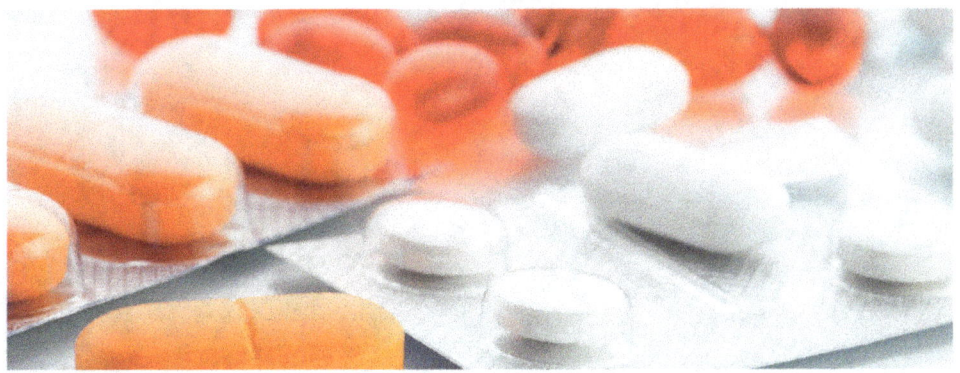

AVOID REFINED CARBOHYDRATES AND FOCUS ON NUTRIENT-DENSE CARBOHYDRATE SOURCES. CARBOHYDRATES FROM VEGETABLES ARE BENEFICIAL TO THE HEALTH AND DIVERSITY OF THE GUT MICROBIOME.

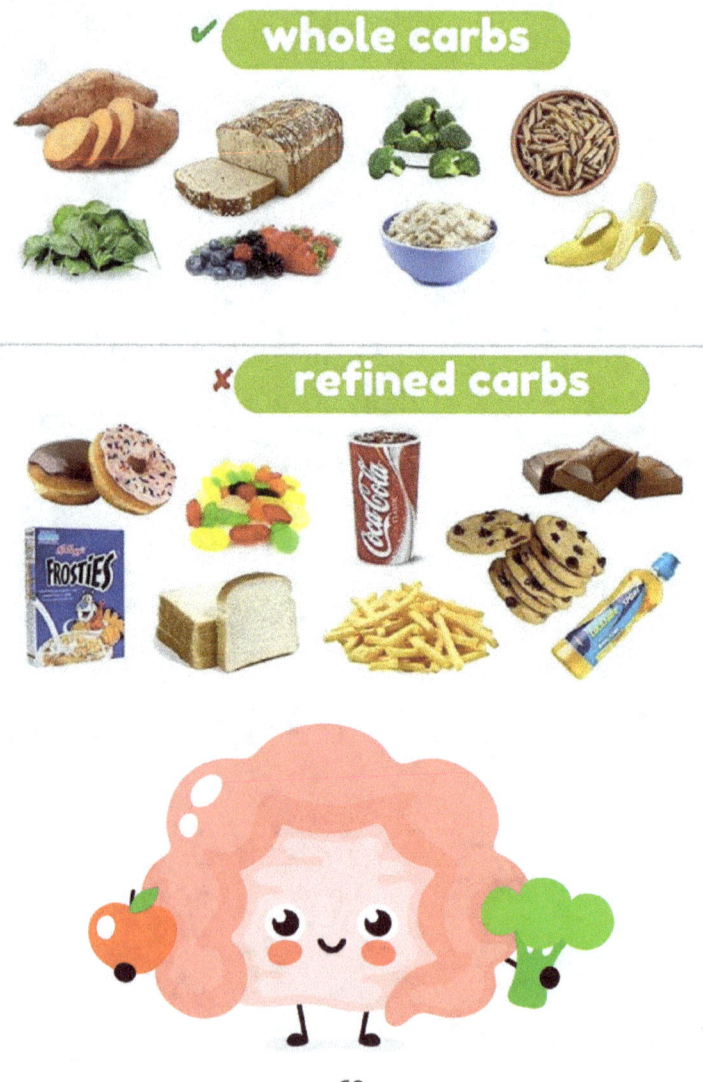

AIM TO AVOID OR REDUCE ALCOHOL CONSUMPTION TO LESS THAN 2 ALCOHOLIC BEVERAGES PER WEEK FOR THE NEXT 8 WEEKS. HIGH ALCOHOL INTAKE CAN HAVE NEGATIVE EFFECTS ON THE DIVERSITY OF THE GUT MICROBIOME.

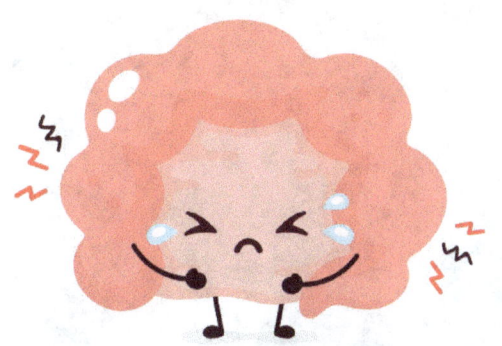
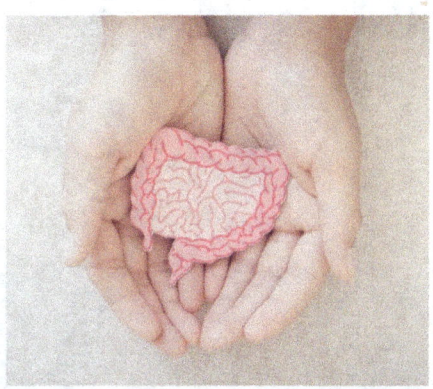
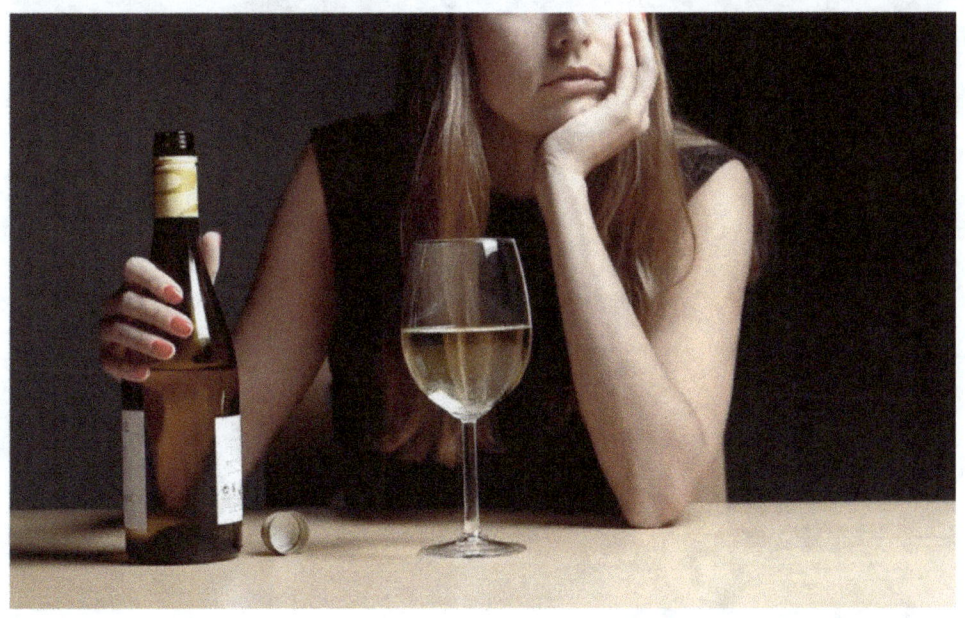

INCREASE WATER AND FLUID INTAKE DEPENDING ON THIRST AND EXERCISE TO SUPPORT DIGESTION AND AVOID DEHYDRATION.

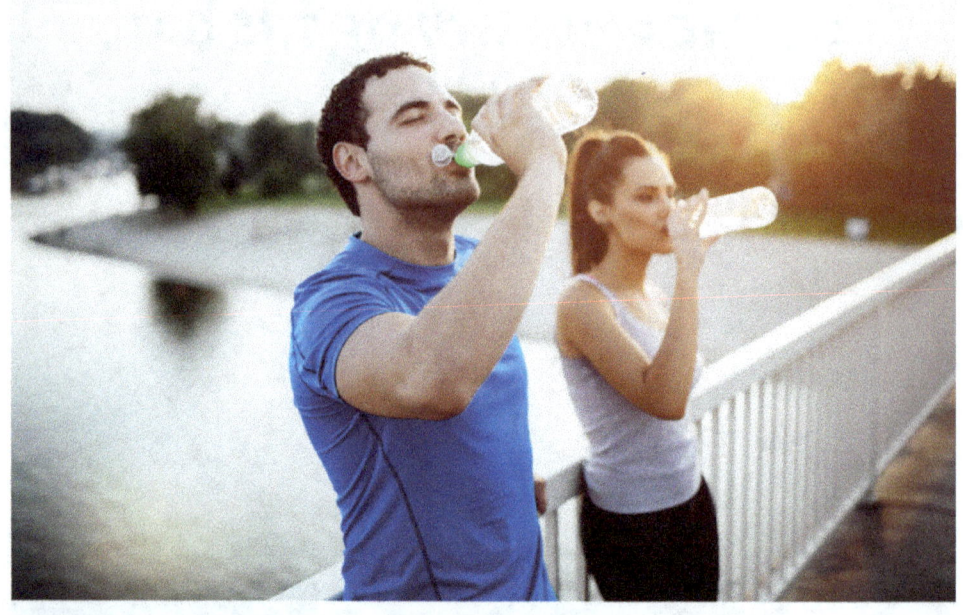
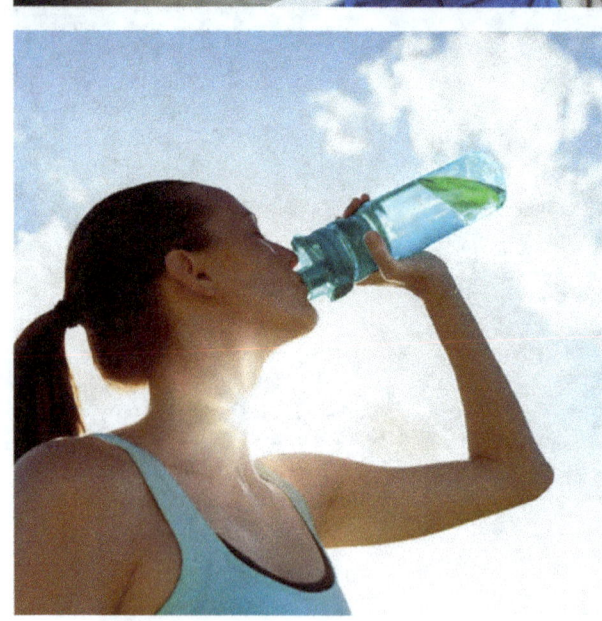
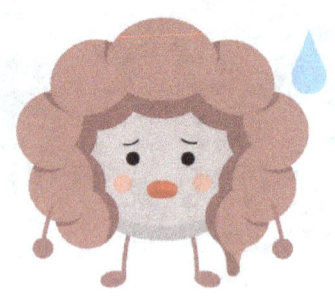

REDUCE CONSUMPTION OF CAFFEINE-CONTAINING PRODUCTS AND LIMIT CAFFEINE CONSUMPTION TO 1-2 CUPS BEFORE NOON. COFFEE CONSUMPTION CAN BE BENEFICIAL TO THE MICROBIOME, BUT EXCESSIVE CONSUMPTION CAN CAUSE DEHYDRATION, IRREGULAR DIGESTION, AND SLEEP DISTURBANCES.

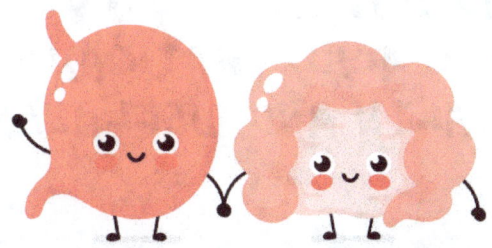

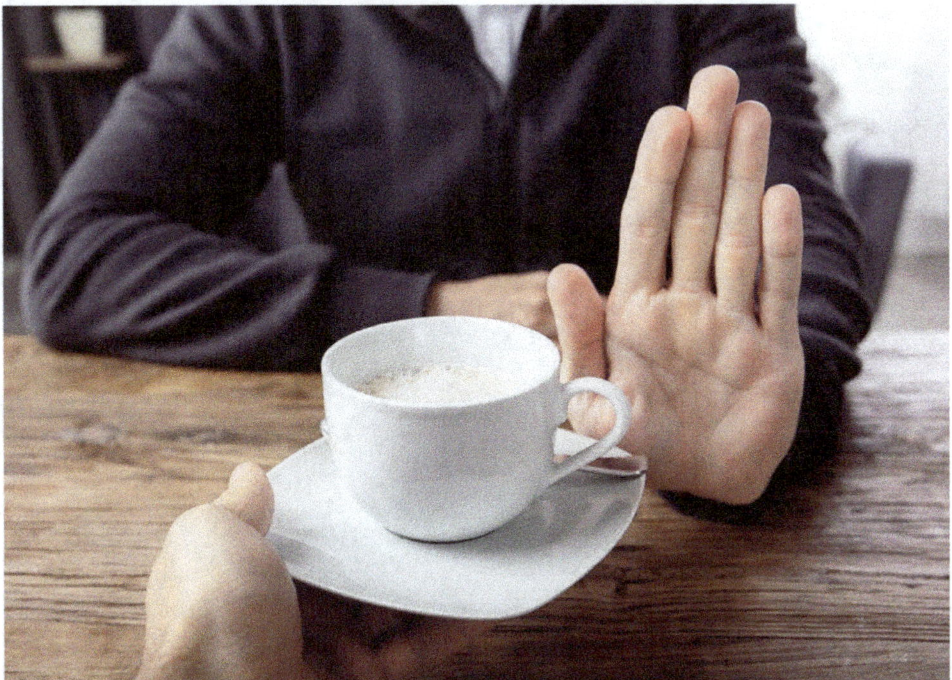

FOCUS ON INCLUDING A VARIETY OF PROTEIN-DENSE FOODS. PROTEIN FROM WHOLE-FOOD SOURCES IS BEST, BUT IT CAN BE BENEFICIAL TO INCLUDE A SUPPLEMENTAL PROTEIN SHAKE, AS NEEDED, TO MEET PROTEIN GOALS. PROTEIN IS MADE UP OF AMINO ACIDS AND AMINO ACIDS ARE USED BY THE GUT BACTERIA TO PRODUCE IMPORTANT METABOLITES, LIKE INDOLE-3-PROPIONIC ACID, THAT CAN SUPPORT HEALTH AND WELLNESS.

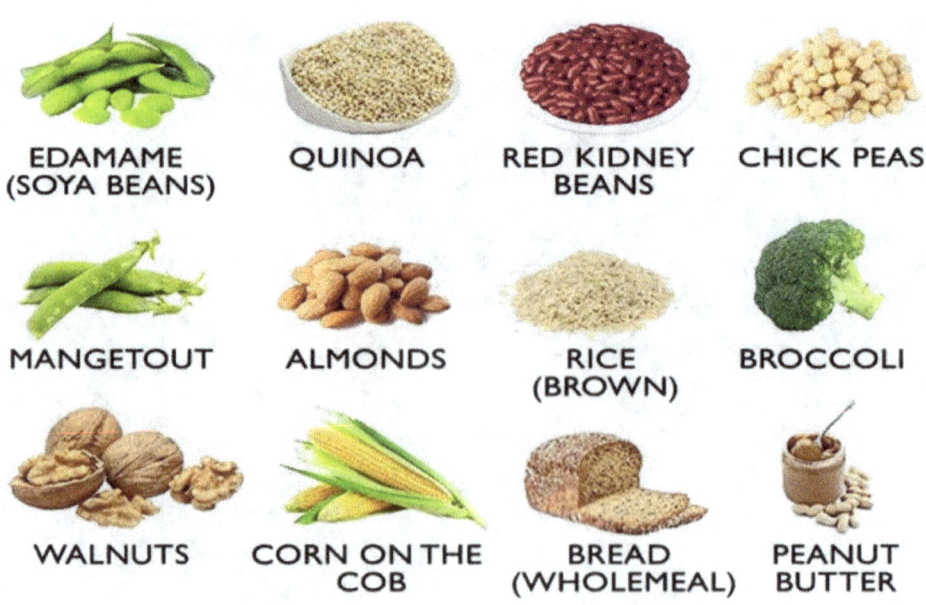

INCORPORATING EITHER PROFESSIONAL MASSAGE OR SELF-MASSAGE WEEKLY CAN STIMULATE NEUROTRANSMITTERS LIKE SEROTONIN, THE PRODUCTION THAT HELPS TO SUPPORT GUT-BRAIN CONNECTION.

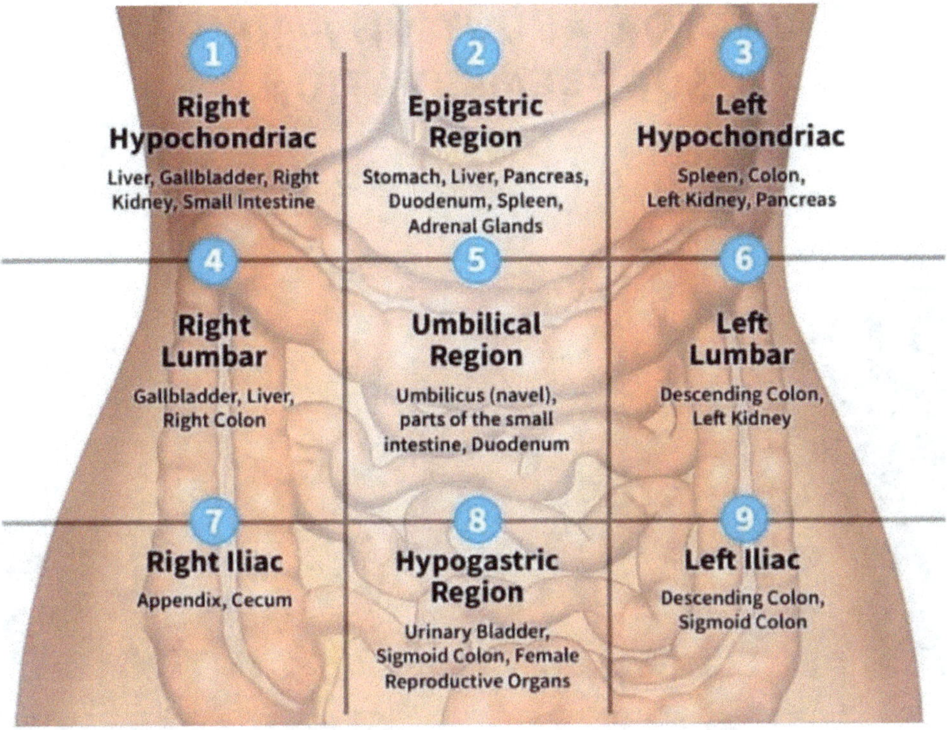

1. Right Hypochondriac — Liver, Gallbladder, Right Kidney, Small Intestine

2. Epigastric Region — Stomach, Liver, Pancreas, Duodenum, Spleen, Adrenal Glands

3. Left Hypochondriac — Spleen, Colon, Left Kidney, Pancreas

4. Right Lumbar — Gallbladder, Liver, Right Colon

5. Umbilical Region — Umbilicus (navel), parts of the small intestine, Duodenum

6. Left Lumbar — Descending Colon, Left Kidney

7. Right Iliac — Appendix, Cecum

8. Hypogastric Region — Urinary Bladder, Sigmoid Colon, Female Reproductive Organs

9. Left Iliac — Descending Colon, Sigmoid Colon

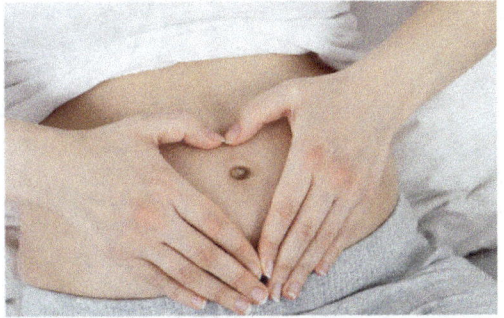
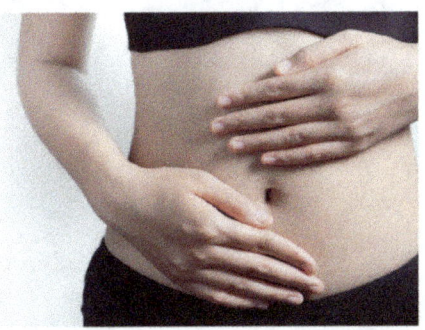

SPENDING AT LEAST 10 MINUTES IN DIRECT SUNLIGHT DAILY CAN BENEFIT VITAMIN PRODUCTION, WHICH HELPS TO SUPPORT THE FUNCTION OF THE GUT MICROBIOME. FOR INDIVIDUALS LIVING IN AN AREA WITH MINIMAL SUN EXPOSURE, CONSIDER TALKING TO YOUR DOCTOR ABOUT VITAMIN D3 SUPPLEMENTATION.

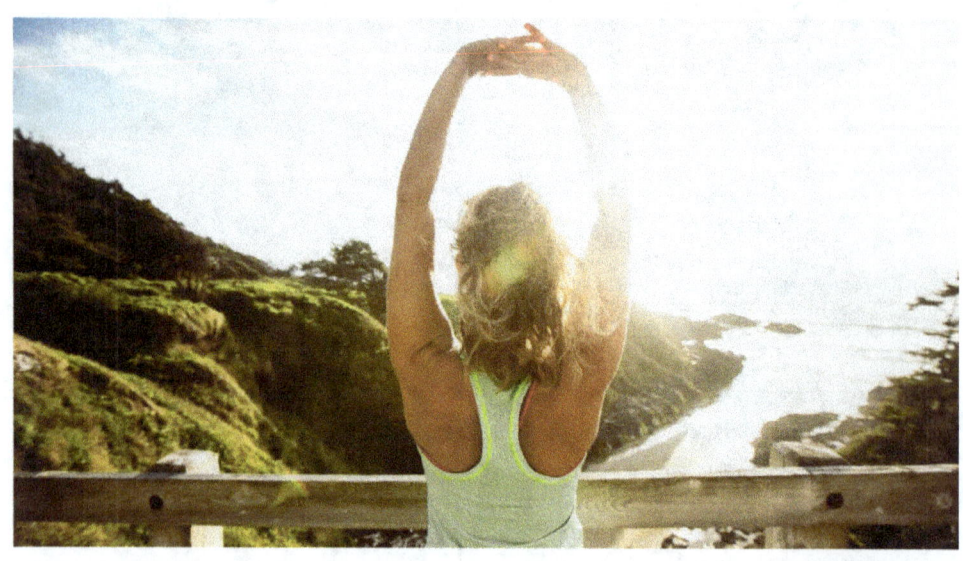

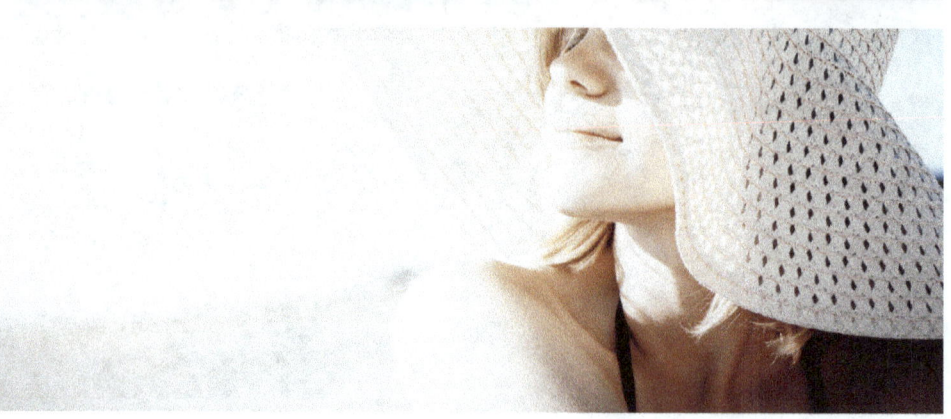

Thank you

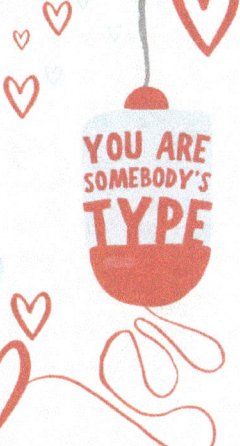

Dear Reader,

I wanted to take a moment to express my sincere gratitude for picking up "Gut Health Hacks." I'm thrilled you've chosen to embark on this journey of understanding and nurturing your gut microbiome. The gut plays a surprisingly powerful role in our overall health, influencing everything from digestion and energy levels to mood and immunity. "Gut Health Hacks" was written with the intention of empowering you to take charge of your gut health with practical, science-backed tips.

Whether you're experiencing specific gut issues or simply looking to optimize your well-being, I hope this book equips you with the knowledge and tools you need. As you delve deeper, don't hesitate to experiment and find what works best for your unique gut.

Thank you again for choosing "Gut Health Hacks." I wish you all the best on your journey to a happier, healthier you, one gut-friendly choice at a time!

www.ingramcontent.com/pod-product-compliance
Lightning Source LLC
Chambersburg PA
CBHW071951210526
45479CB00003B/891